2 -

Primary Care Provider's
Guide to Cardiology

Primary Care Provider's Guide to Cardiology

Editors

Glenn N. Levine, M.D.
Assistant Professor of Medicine
Baylor College of Medicine
Co-Director, Cardiac Catheter-
  ization Laboratory
Houston V. A. Medical Center
Houston, Texas

Douglas L. Mann, M.D.
Professor of Medicine
Baylor College of Medicine
Chief, Section of Cardiology
Houston V. A. Medical Center
Houston, Texas

 LIPPINCOTT WILLIAMS & WILKINS
A **Wolters Kluwer** Company
Philadelphia · Baltimore · New York · London
Buenos Aires · Hong Kong · Sydney · Tokyo

Acquisitions Editor: Timothy Y. Hiscock
Development Editor: Leah Ann Kiehne Hayes
Manufacturing Manager: Kevin Watt
Supervising Editor: Mary Ann McLaughlin
Production Service: Colophon
Cover Designer: Joan Greenfield
Compositor: Circle Graphics
Printer: Vicks Litho

Printed in the USA

Library of Congress Cataloging-in-Publication Data

Primary care provider's guide to cardiology / editors, Glenn N. Levine, Douglas L. Mann.
   p.   cm.
  Includes bibliographical references and index.
  ISBN 0-683-30688-X (alk. paper)
  1. Cardiology. 2. Primary care (Medicine) 3. Heart—Diseases—Treatment. I. Levine,
Glenn N. II. Mann, D.
  [DNLM: 1. Cardiovascular Diseases. WG 120 P9525 2000]
  RC667.P75 2000
  616.1′2—dc21

                              99-042866

10 9 8 7 6 5 4 3 2 1

To my faithful friend and companion for all these years, Daisy D.
GLENN N. LEVINE

To my family, Stephanie, Jonathan, Erica and especially Laura
DOUGLAS L. MANN

Contents

Foreword

In today's continually changing medical and economic environments, the health care profession is witnessing a shift in the care for many patients with cardiovascular disease from the specialist to the primary care provider. This shift has been driven by multiple factors, including a renewed emphasis on primary care, the inexorable push for more outpatient treatment and shorter hospital stays, and the ever-present consideration of lowering the overall cost of health care. Given this shifting landscape, the primary care provider will be called upon to assume the management of patients with cardiovascular conditions to an increasingly greater degree in the ensuing years.

In the *Primary Care Provider's Guide to Cardiology,* the editors have developed a relatively simple "how to" reference source that provides diagnostic and management guidelines for most of the common cardiac conditions seen in routine clinical practice, including congestive heart failure, hypercholesterolemia, atrial fibrillation, unstable angina, and myocardial infarction. This book gives the primary care provider clinically relevant information presented in a concise and cogent manner. Moreover, this information is presented in a manner that should be easy to follow and apply. The utilization of multiple tables and algorithms enhances the user-friendly aspects of the book. I believe that this book should serve as an important addition to the primary care provider's armamentarium of "readable" reference sources to help with his/her increasing role in the diagnosis and management of patients with a broad variety of cardiovascular problems. I recommend it enthusiastically!

James T. Willerson, M.D.
Edward Randall III Professor and Chairman
Department of Internal Medicine
University of Texas Health Sciences Center at Houston
Medical Director, Chief of Cardiology, Director of Cardiology Research
*   and Co-Director*
Cullen Cardiovascular Research Laboratories at the Texas Heart Institute
Chief and Chair of Cardiology, St. Luke's Episcopal Hospital
Chief of Medical Services at Hermann Memorial Hospital

Preface

In this changing medical environment, primary care providers will increasingly be managing patients with common cardiac conditions. While we have found that there are a plethora of "mini-textbooks" on cardiology, there is no book that is specifically focused on the evaluation and treatment of common cardiac conditions. We have therefore set out to write a "how to" manual for primary care providers that provides concise, easily understandable, and clinically relevant information on the appropriate management of patients with cardiac conditions that primary care providers will encounter both in the outpatient and inpatient settings. We have striven to utilize tables, figures, and algorithms as much as possible to present and summarize management guidelines in a user-friendly manner. We have also taken care to include only information that is clinically relevant so that each chapter can be quickly read in five to ten minutes, thus ensuring that the book truly can serve as a "quick reference" to the busy practitioner. Finally, we have also included "clinical pearls" that we believe provide additional relevant information for the primary care provider regarding patient care. We hope that this book proves to be a useful resource to you in the care of patients with cardiac diseases.

Glenn N. Levine, M.D.
Douglas L. Mann, M.D.

Contributing Authors

M. Nadir Ali, M.B.B.S
Assistant Professor of Medicine
Baylor College of Medicine
Director, Cardiac Catheterization Laboratory
Houston V. A. Medical Center
2002 Holcombe Boulevard
Houston, Texas 77030

Karen M. Belco, B.S.N., R.N.
Device Specialist
Cardiology Associates of Lubbock
3514 21st Street
Lubbock, Texas 79410

Sheilah Bernard, M.D.
Associate Clinical Professor of Medicine
Boston University School of Medicine
Director of Cardiology Ambulatory Services
Section of Cardiology
Boston Medical Center
1 Boston Medical Center Place, C-8
Boston, Massachusetts 02118

Alvin Blaustein, M.D.
Associate Professor of Medicine
Baylor College of Medicine
Director, Non-invasive Laboratory
Houston V. A. Medical Center
2002 Holcombe Blvd
Houston, Texas 77030

Richard I. Fogel, M.D.
Northside Cardiology Care Associates
8333 Naab Road, Suite 200
Indianapolis, Indiana 46260

Glenn N. Levine, M.D.
Assistant Professor of Medicine
Baylor College of Medicine
Co-Director, Cardiac Catheterization Laboratory
Houston V. A. Medical Center
2002 Holcombe Boulevard
Houston, Texas 77030

Douglas L. Mann, M.D.
Professor of Medicine
Baylor College of Medicine
Chief, Section of Cardiology
Houston V. A. Medical Center
2002 Holcombe Boulevard
Houston, Texas 77030

W. Robb MacLellan, M.D.
Assistant Professor of Medicine and Physiology
University of California, Los Angeles School of Medicine
675 C.E. Young Drive, MRL 3-645
Los Angeles, California 90095

Sherif F. Nagueh, M.D.
Assistant Professor of Medicine
Baylor College of Medicine
Section of Cardiology
Methodist Hospital
6536 Fannin
Houston, Texas 77030

Jaggarao S. Nattama, M.D.
Assistant Professor of Medicine,
Baylor College of Medicine
Director, Electrophysiology and Pacing
Houston V. A. Medical Center
2002 Holcombe Boulevard
Houston, Texas 77030

Niraj Varma, M.D., M.R.C.P.
Assistant Professor of Medicine
Case Western Reserve University
Division of Cardiology
University Hospital of Cleveland
11100 Euclid Avenue
Cleveland, Ohio 44106

1

Evaluation and Management of the Patient with Congestive Heart Failure

Glenn N. Levine and *Douglas L. Mann

*Baylor College of Medicine, Cardiac Catheterization Laboratory,
Section of Cardiology, Houston V. A. Medical Center, Houston, Texas 77030

Four million Americans alone have been diagnosed with "congestive heart failure." Approximately 400,000 new cases of heart failure are diagnosed annually in the United States, and it is expected that one of ten Americans over the age of 70 years will develop heart failure. Therefore, it is important for primary care practitioners to be comfortable with the evaluation and management of the patient with heart failure. In this chapter, the steps in the evaluation of a patient who presents with signs and symptoms of heart failure will be outlined, and the approach to the management of patients with congestive heart failure will be discussed.

INITIAL STEPS IN THE EVALUATION OF THE PATIENT WHO PRESENTS WITH CONGESTIVE HEART FAILURE

The initial office or hospital evaluation of the patient who presents with signs and symptoms of heart failure should include a directed history, the physical examination, electrocardiography, and chest radiography.

History

The history should include questions regarding symptoms of congestive heart failure, including dyspnea on exertion, orthopnea (needing to elevate the head with pillows while sleeping), paroxysmal nocturnal dyspnea (where the patient wakes up at night short of breath), and lower extremity edema.

Physical Examination

The physical examination should include assessment for jugular venous distention (indicative of elevated right heart pressures) and pulmonary rales (indicative of elevated left heart pressures), evaluation of the heart's point of maximum impulse (which often is displaced inferolaterally in patients with dilated and poorly contractile left ventricles), the presence of systolic or diastolic murmurs, and the presence of an S3 gallop.

Electrocardiography

The electrocardiogram should be examined for signs of left ventricular hypertrophy and/or abnormalities suggesting coronary artery disease (such as old Q waves).

Chest Radiography

The chest x-ray film should be examined for evidence of pulmonary vascular congestion and pulmonary edema, pleural effusions, and heart size (because a large heart seen on chest x-ray film correlates with a dilated and poorly contractile left ventricle).

DISTINGUISHING WHETHER CONGESTIVE HEART FAILURE IS DUE TO SYSTOLIC DYSFUNCTION OR DIASTOLIC DYSFUNCTION

Because the signs and symptoms of congestive heart failure may arise from abnormalities of either ventricular contraction or ventricular relaxation and the treatment of these two abnormalities is completely different, the primary care practitioner must be able to understand these two disease processes and be able to distinguish between them. In patients with abnormalities of ventricular contraction, the ability of the left ventricle to contract is impaired, and the ventricle is not able to pump enough blood out of the ventricle and to muscles and organs. This commonly is referred to as "systolic dysfunction." In patients with impaired ventricular relaxation, a stiff, often thickened left ventricle is not able to "relax" in diastole. Because of this impaired ability to relax, filling pressures in the left ventricle during diastole are elevated. In diastole, when the mitral valve is open, pressures in the left ventricle are reflected back into the left atrium and pulmonary circulation. The lungs "see" these elevated pressures and become congested. This abnormality commonly is referred to as "diastolic dysfunction."

As noted earlier, both systolic dysfunction and diastolic dysfunction can lead to symptoms such as dyspnea and signs of heart failure such as rales on examination and pulmonary vascular congestion on chest x-ray film. Therefore, the most important step in the evaluation of the patient who presents with congestive heart failure is to distinguish if the heart failure is due to systolic or diastolic dysfunction. This is done by assessing left ventricular ejection fraction. Left ventricular ejection fraction can be assessed noninvasively by either echocardiography or radionuclide ventriculography (gated blood pool scan or multiple gated acquisition). The cardiac echocardiogram allows one to obtain additional important information, particularly whether there are any significant valvular abnormalities, and it is the study of choice among most cardiologists.

In general, if left ventricular ejection fraction is depressed (less than 40%) and there are no significant valvular abnormalities that could be causing the heart failure (such as aortic stenosis or mitral regurgitation), the patient's heart failure can be attributed to left ventricular systolic dysfunction. Alternately, if the ejection fraction is greater than 40%, one should consider the diagnosis of diastolic dysfunction. The steps in the evaluation of the patient with congestive heart failure are summarized in Fig. 1.1. In the remainder of this chapter, management of the patient with systolic dysfunction and congestive heart failure is discussed.

SELECTING MEDICATIONS FOR THE TREATMENT OF SYSTOLIC DYSFUNCTION AND CONGESTIVE HEART FAILURE

The goals of medical therapy are to (i) improve the quality of life, (ii) avoid the need for future hospitalizations, and (iii) prolong life. Medications now available to the primary care provider make it possible to achieve all three

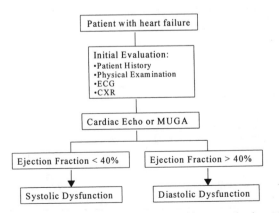

FIG. 1.1. Steps in the evaluation of the patient with congestive heart failure.

of these goals. The basic classes of drugs that are used to treat patients with systolic dysfunction and heart failure are listed in Table 1.1.

In general, patients with left ventricular dysfunction and only minimal or mild symptoms of heart failure (New York Heart Association [NYHA] class I or II) should be treated with digoxin and angiotensin-converting enzyme (ACE) inhibitors. Use of diuretics should be avoided in these patients because of the risk of dehydration and activation of the renin-angiotensin system (which can lead to disease progression and worsening of symptoms). Patients with left ventricular dysfunction and moderate or severe symptoms (NYHA class III or IV) should be treated with diuretics, digoxin, and ACE inhibitors. In patients who are unable to tolerate ACE inhibitors (due to the development of renal failure, symptomatic hypotension, severe nonproductive cough, or angioedema), the combination of hydralazine and isosorbide dinitrate (Isordil) should be used instead. The drugs used in the treatment of heart failure are discussed in the following.

Diuretics

Diuretics primarily serve to relieve symptoms of heart failure due to volume overload. In patients with milder volume overload, the less potent diuretic hydrochlorothiazide (HCTZ) can be utilized. The starting dose of HCTZ is 25 mg daily, and it can be increased as needed up to a maximum dose of 50 mg daily. In patients with more severe volume overload or in those who do not respond to HCTZ, furosemide (Lasix) should be used. Lasix should be initiated at a dose of 10 to 20 mg daily. The dose can be increased as needed up to a maximum dose of 160 mg b.i.d.

Digoxin

Digoxin can improve heart failure symptoms and recently has been shown to decrease the incidence of future hospitalizations. The starting dose in

TABLE 1.1. *Classes of medications used in the treatment of congestive heart failure and their clinical benefits*

Class of drug	Improve symptoms	Prevent hospitalizations	Prolong life
Diuretics	Yes	?	No
Digoxin	Yes	Yes	No
ACE inhibitors	Yes	Yes	Yes
Hydralazine/isordil	Yes	Yes	Yes
Angiotensin receptor blockers	?Yes	?Yes	?Yes
Beta blockers	No	Yes	Yes

ACE, angiotensin-converting enzyme.

most patients is 0.125 mg p.o. daily. Serum levels should be checked after 4 to 5 days of therapy, and the daily dose should be titrated to achieve a serum digoxin concentration of 1.0 to 2.0 mg/dL.

◆ CLINICAL PEARLS ◆

Digoxin is renally excreted, and the dose needs to be decreased in patients with renal insufficiency. The usual dose in patients with renal failure who are on dialysis is 0.125 mg p.o. every other day.

Angiotensin-converting Enzyme Inhibitors

Angiotensin-converting enzyme inhibitors have been shown in multiple studies to not only improve the symptoms of congestive heart failure and decrease the need for future hospitalizations, but also to prolong life. Thus, their use has become the standard of care in patients with systolic dysfunction and heart failure. Many ACE inhibitors now are available. The starting doses, recommended target doses, and maximum doses for these ACE inhibitors are listed in Table 1.2.

◆ CLINICAL PEARLS ◆

Because ACE inhibitors can interfere with and/or impair renal function, patients' blood urea nitrogen (BUN), creatinine, and potassium levels should be monitored during the first several weeks of therapy. Mild increases in BUN and/or creatinine should be tolerated. However, significant increases in BUN and/or creatinine, or the occurrence of hyperkalemia, are indications to discontinue ACE inhibitor therapy.

TABLE 1.2. *Commonly used ACE inhibitors and the recommended starting dose, target dose for the treatment of congestive heart failure, and maximum dose*

Medication	Initial dose	Target dose	Maximum dose
Captopril (Capoten)	6.25 mg t.i.d.	50 mg t.i.d.	100 mg t.i.d.
Enalopril (Vasotec)	2.5 mg b.i.d.	10 mg b.i.d.	20 mg b.i.d.
Fosinopril (Monopril)	10 mg q.d.	20 mg q.d.	40 mg q.d.
Linisopril (Primivil, Zestril)	5 mg q.d.	20 mg q.d.	40 mg q.d.
Quinapril (Accupril)	10 mg q.d.	40 mg q.d.	80 mg q.d.

Brand names are given in parentheses.
ACE, angiotensin-converting enzyme.

Hydralazine and Isosorbide Dinitrate

The combination of hydralazine and isosorbide dinitrate has been shown, like ACE inhibitors, to prolong life, although hydralazine and isosorbide dinitrate is not as effective as ACE inhibitor therapy. Thus, although ACE inhibitors remain the first-line therapy for patients with congestive heart failure, those patients unable to tolerate ACE inhibitors should be treated with hydralazine and isosorbide dinitrate. Hydralazine should be started at a dose of 10 to 25 mg t.i.d. and titrated to a target dose of 75 mg t.i.d. Isosorbide dinitrate should be started at a dose of 10 mg t.i.d. and titrated up to a target dose of 40 mg t.i.d.

Angiotensin Receptor Antagonists

Drugs that block the type I angiotensin receptor, often referred to as angiotensin receptor blockers, represent a relatively new and emerging class of drugs for treating patients with heart failure. At present, angiotensin receptor antagonists have not been definitively shown to prolong life and prevent hospitalization in patients with advanced heart failure, although there are several suggestive studies. Therefore, at present these drugs should not be used instead of ACE inhibitors as first-line therapy in heart failure patients. However, many people now advocate the use of angiotensin receptor blockers in patients who are ACE intolerant.

Beta Blockers

Beta blockers with ancillary vasodilating properties (e.g., carvedilol) have been shown to prolong life in patients with mild-to-moderate heart failure who were already receiving conventional therapy for heart failure. However, unlike ACE inhibitors, which are relatively well tolerated, beta blockers can transiently worsen heart failure. Therefore, it is absolutely imperative that these agents be started at the lowest dose possible and then titrated up on a weekly or every other week basis.

Currently, the only beta blocker that is approved for use in heart failure is carvedilol, which should be started at a dose of 3.125 mg b.i.d. and then gradually titrated up to a final dose of 25 mg b.i.d. At the time of this writing, metoprolol also has been shown in one large trial to be beneficial in patients with heart failure (although at this time it is not yet approved by the Food and Drug Administration for this indication). Metoprolol should be started at a dose of 25 mg q.d., increased to 25 mg b.i.d. after 1 to 2 weeks, and then gradually titrated up to a final target dose (if tolerated) of 100 mg b.i.d.

Beta blockers should not be used in patients with bradycardia, first-degree heart block, or significant obstructive lung disease or pulmonary edema. Because administration of beta blockers can lead to transient hypotension, these patients should be observed in the primary care provider's office for at least 1 hour after the beta-blocker dose is increased to ensure that the patient will tolerate the drug.

Transient worsening of heart failure generally is treated easily by an increase in diuretics rather than a decrease in the dose of beta blockers; however, for beta-blocker–induced heart failure that is unresponsive to diuretics, the patient may need to be titrated down to a more acceptable dose. Rarely is it necessary to completely stop administration of the beta blocker.

CONSIDERATIONS IN THE TREATMENT OF VENTRICULAR ECTOPY AND VENTRICULAR ARRHYTHMIAS

Sudden cardiac death accounts for up to 40% of all deaths in patients with congestive heart failure. Thus, management decisions regarding ventricular arrhythmias is an important part of the routine care of patients with heart failure. Unfortunately, medical therapy has proved less than optimal in improving patient outcome. Further, all antiarrhythmic drugs, with the exception of amiodarone, have "proarrhythmic" actions (i.e., they can precipitate arrhythmias).

Premature Ventricular Contractions

There is no evidence that treatment of premature ventricular contractions improves outcome in patients with congestive heart failure. Given this and the fact that all antiarrhythmic drugs have side effects (including proarrhythmic effects), attempts at suppression of premature ventricular contractions with medications is not recommended in these patients.

Nonsustained Ventricular Tachycardia

Nonsustained ventricular tachycardia (NSVT) is a catch-all phrase that can refer to a run of ventricular ectopy as short as three beats in a row or as long as 30 to 60 seconds. In patients with NSVT who have no symptoms, no treatment strategy has been shown to be superior to no treatment at all. In patients with symptomatic NSVT (such as the development of lightheadedness or frank syncope), antiarrhythmic therapy (often amiodarone 200 to 400 mg daily) or automatic implantable cardiac defibrillator implantation should be initiated. Therefore, referral to an electrophysiologist should be considered in these patients.

✪ CLINICAL PEARLS ✪

Because of the multiple toxicities of amiodarone, patients taking this antiarrhythmic drug should undergo chest radiography (to screen for interstitial fibrosis), liver function tests (to test for hepatitis), and thyroid function tests (to test for hyperthyroidism or hypothyroidism) every 6 months.

Sustained Ventricular Tachycardia

Patients with sustained ventricular tachycardia (usually defined as ventricular tachycardia lasting more than 30 to 60 seconds) are at high risk of sudden death. Most patients will be managed with automatic implantable cardioverter defibrillator implantation; thus, these patients should be referred to an electrophysiologist.

CONSIDERATIONS IN DECIDING WHETHER TO ANTICOAGULATE THE PATIENT WITH LEFT VENTRICULAR DYSFUNCTION AND CONGESTIVE HEART FAILURE

In the past, it was common practice to anticoagulate patients with dilated cardiomyopathies and congestive heart failure. However, recent studies have revealed that there is little, if any, benefit in anticoagulating all such patients. Therefore, in general, it is now recommended that most such patients not be anticoagulated. Anticoagulation (at an international normalized ratio of 2.0 to 3.0) is recommended in patients with congestive heart failure who also have either atrial fibrillation or are found to have a mobile left ventricular thrombus on cardiac echocardiogram.

LIFESTYLE RECOMMENDATIONS FOR HEART FAILURE PATIENTS

Dietary Restrictions

One of the most frequently overlooked problems in managing patients with advanced heart failure are issues regarding dietary restrictions. It is recommended that all patients with congestive heart failure be referred to a nutritionist for review of the proper diet, which includes sodium restriction to 2 to 3 g per day and a low fat/low cholesterol diet in those with concurrent coronary artery disease.

Fluid Restrictions

Fluid restriction is only useful in patients who become hyponatremic (low serum sodium level) during heart failure treatment (particularly diuretic therapy). In patients with hyponatremia, fluid intake should be restricted to 1 liter per day.

Alcohol

Alcohol intake generally should be limited to one drink per day and no more than two drinks per day. In patients with a cardiomyopathy believed due to excess alcohol intake, any and all use of alcohol is contraindicated.

Exercise

In patients with minimal-to-moderate heart failure symptoms (NYHA class I to III), moderate aerobic exercise programs (walking, light bicycling, swimming) should be encouraged. In patients with severe symptoms (NYHA class IV), exercise (other than simple walking) is not recommended.

SUMMARY

Appropriate treatment for patients with heart failure secondary to depressed left ventricular function can improve quality of life, prevent future hospitalizations, and prolong life. Selection of medications and, to some extent, lifestyle recommendations depend on the severity of patients' symptoms. Patients with significant ventricular arrhythmias should be considered for referral to electrophysiologists.

2

Approach to the Patient with Syncope

Richard I. Fogel and *Niraj Varma

*Northside Cardiology Care Associates, Indianapolis, Indiana 46260;
and *Division of Cardiology, Case Western Reserve University,
University Hospital of Cleveland, Cleveland, Ohio 44106*

Syncope is a transient loss of consciousness. It is a common symptom seen in clinical practice, accounting for 3% of all emergency room visits. One third to one half of the population will experience a syncopal event at some point. Determining the exact cause of the syncopal event often is difficult. However, appropriate evaluation of a patient is crucial, because some causes of syncope are benign and carry an excellent prognosis, whereas other causes, especially those due to cardiovascular disease, are associated with a high rate of 1-year mortality. In this chapter, an organized approach to the patient with syncope is discussed.

CARDIAC CAUSES OF SYNCOPE

The many etiologies of syncope can be usefully divided into cardiac and noncardiac causes (Table 2.1). Cardiac causes can be further subdivided into arrhythmias and mechanical obstructions.

Arrhythmias

Arrhythmic causes of syncope are very important to identify, as they often are life threatening yet are responsive to treatment. Bradyarrhythmias, such as sick sinus syndrome and high-grade atrioventricular (AV) block, can be treated with implantation of a permanent pacemaker. However, before proceeding to permanent pacemaker implantation, the care provider should exclude reversible causes of bradycardia such as bradycardia associated with beta-adrenergic blocking agents, as well as the calcium channel blockers verapamil and diltiazem.

TABLE 2.1. *Cardiac and noncardiac causes of syncope*

Cardiac causes
   I. Arrhythmic
      A. Bradyarrhythmia
         Sick sinus syndrome
         Atrioventricular nodal block
      B. Tachyarrhythmias
         Supraventricular tachycardia
         Ventricular tachycardia
  II. Mechanical
      A. Aortic stenosis
      B. Hypertrophic cardiomyopathy
      C. Atrial myxoma
      D. Pulmonary embolism
Noncardiac Causes
   I. Neurocardiogenic (vasovagal) syncope
  II. Orthostatic hypotension
      A. Neuropathy
      B. Volume depletion or anemia
      C. Drug induced (e.g., alpha-adrenergic blocking agents)
  III. Carotid sinus hypersensitivity
  IV. Neurologic conditions
      A. Vertebrobasilar disease
      B. Seizures
   V. Toxic and metabolic causes (e.g., hypoglycemia)

Tachyarrhythmias can be either supraventricular or ventricular. Although supraventricular tachycardia most commonly produces intense palpitations, the sudden onset of a rapid tachycardia can result in a marked fall in blood pressure and presyncope.

Ventricular tachycardia is the most concerning arrhythmia, as it is a common mechanism of death. It occurs most commonly in patients with a history of myocardial infarction or in those with dilated cardiomyopathy. The adage that the only difference between syncope and sudden cardiac death is that patients with syncope regain consciousness may be most relevant to patients with ventricular tachycardia. Fortunately, once ventricular tachycardia is identified, excellent therapeutic options are available.

Mechanical Obstructions

The most common cardiac mechanical obstruction that can cause syncope is aortic stenosis, which should be suspected in any elderly patient, especially if the syncopal episode is associated with exertion. In younger patients, a dynamic obstruction most commonly will be attributable to hypertrophic cardiomyopathy. In this syndrome, states of increased left ventricular contractility can result in systolic anterior motion of the mitral valve, dynamic outflow tract obstruction, and syncope. The finding of a murmur that increases with the Valsalva maneuver in a young person is highly suggestive of hypertrophic cardiomyopathy. Rarer causes of obstructed blood flow that can lead to syncope include atrial myxomas and pulmonary embolism.

NONCARDIAC CAUSES OF SYNCOPE

Several noncardiac causes of syncope should be considered in the patient who presents with or describes one or more episodes of syncope (Table 2.1).

Neurocardiogenic Syncope

Neurocardiogenic syncope, also called vasovagal or vasodepressor syncope, is the most common cause of syncope in otherwise healthy individuals. It is caused by a neurologic reflex, which leads to peripheral vasodilation that is not compensated for by a rise in cardiac output, leading to a fall in blood pressure and cerebral hypoperfusion. Precipitating factors include pain, emotional stress, and fear. Syncope often is preceded by prodromal symptoms such as nausea, diaphoresis, dizziness, and blurred vision. Neurocardiogenic syncope is a relatively benign condition with an excellent long-term prognosis.

Orthostatic Hypotension

The term orthostatic hypotension refers to the phenomenon in which blood pressure drops when a person who has been supine or sitting suddenly stands up. It results from a decrease in venous return to the heart, with a resultant decrease in cardiac output. There also may be a failure of reflex mechanisms that ordinarily would maintain blood pressure. Orthostatic hypotension may occur in those who are taking diuretics, are severely anemic, or are volume depleted. It also may occur in patients taking medications that cause arterial vasodilation (particularly the alpha-receptor blocking agents used in the treatment of benign prostatic hypertrophy) and in patients with autonomic neuropathies such as diabetes. The diagnosis is based on the blood pressure and heart rate measurements taken with the patient in the supine, sitting, and standing positions.

Carotid Sinus Hypersensitivity

Carotid sinus hypersensitivity is the cause of syncope in many elderly patients. It may be precipitated by tight collars or ties, neck movement, or other processes that can affect the carotid baroreceptors. Diagnosis is derived in part from carotid sinus massage (if no carotid bruits are present) and observing a pause of more than 3 seconds during continuous electrocardiogram (ECG) monitoring, a dramatic fall in blood pressure, or both.

Neurologic Conditions

Although often suspected, neurologic disease is an uncommon cause of syncope. Carotid disease results in hemispheric symptoms such as hemiparesis, but it is unlikely to depress consciousness. Posterior circulation disease (i.e., vertebral artery disease), however, can cause syncope if the brainstem reticular activating system is involved. We have found that the usual "shotgun" neurologic evaluation, which includes computed tomography, electroencephalography, and carotid ultrasound, frequently is not useful unless the patient's history strongly suggests seizures or vertebral basilar insufficiency.

INITIAL STEPS IN THE EVALUATION OF THE PATIENT WITH SYNCOPE

The history, physical examination, and ECG can provide important clues about the etiology of syncope and are diagnostic in approximately 50% of patients.

History

A cardiac tachyarrhythmia should be suspected if there is an abrupt loss of consciousness without any prodrome or if syncope is preceded by palpitations. Prodromal symptoms such as nausea and diaphoresis often precede neurocardiogenic syncope. The care provider should determine if the patient has a history of cardiac disease, particularly previous myocardial infarction or known cardiomyopathy. These conditions are associated with a much higher risk of ventricular tachyarrhythmias. The care provider should inquire about any family history of unexplained or sudden cardiac death, because such a history may suggest hypertrophic cardiomyopathy (which can be familial).

Physical Examination

Physical examination is most helpful in establishing the presence of structural heart disease. Supine and standing blood pressures taken 3 to 5 minutes apart can facilitate diagnosis of orthostatic hypotension. The presence of cardiac murmurs suggests valvular disease or hypertrophic cardiomyopathy. After auscultation for carotid bruits, the patient should receive carotid sinus massage on one side at a time with continuous ECG monitoring. Replication of presyncope or syncopal symptoms with carotid sinus massage and induced bradycardia indicates carotid sinus hypersensitivity.

Electrocardiogram

The 12-lead ECG is an essential component of the syncope evaluation. The presence of an old myocardial infarction or a bundle branch block can yield diagnostic clues to the etiology of syncope and suggest the need for further electrophysiologic assessment. The presence of high-grade AV block, especially if correlated with symptoms, indicates the need for permanent pacemaker implantation. The ECG can indicate prolonged QT syndrome and ventricular preexcitation (i.e., Wolff-Parkinson-White syndrome), which are two important causes of syncope in patients with otherwise structurally normal hearts.

Other Initial Evaluation

When a cardiac etiology of syncope is suspected, the care provider should obtain an echocardiogram. Although the test is rarely diagnostic (unless aortic stenosis or hypertrophic cardiomyopathy is identified), the presence of a normal echocardiographic evaluation and normal ECG usually suggests a noncardiac cause of syncope and a more benign prognosis.

❖ CLINICAL PEARLS ❖

Establishing—or ruling out—a cardiovascular etiology of syncope is critical, because a high rate of mortality is associated with cardiovascular causes of syncope.

SUBSEQUENT EVALUATION

Despite a thorough evaluation including history, physical examination, and ECG, approximately 50% of patients will not have a clear diagnosis. The initial goal of a subsequent evaluation is to identify the etiology of the syncope. A secondary goal of this evaluation, even if no clear etiology can be determined, is to rule out a cardiac cause, particularly tachyarrhythmia, because cardiac causes are associated with higher morbidity, whereas noncardiac causes are associated with a more benign prognosis. One approach to this subsequent evaluation is shown in Fig. 2.1. and presented in the following discussion.

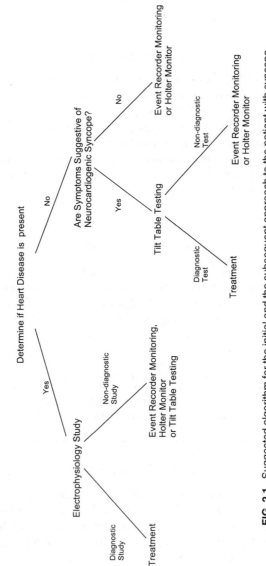

FIG. 2.1. Suggested algorithm for the initial and the subsequent approach to the patient with syncope.

Evaluation of Patients with Structural Heart Disease: Electrophysiologic Testing

In patients with evidence of structural (or electrical) heart disease, inpatient evaluation and referral to an electrophysiologist for electrophysiologic testing are indicated.

◦ CLINICAL PEARLS ◦

Electrophysiologic testing involves the placement of catheters through the femoral vein under fluoroscopic guidance into the heart. Testing of sinus node function and AV conduction can be accomplished. Additionally, through programmed stimulation of the ventricle, it can be determined whether ventricular tachycardia can be induced.

Important prognostic and therapeutic information can be obtained, and the test is diagnostic in approximately 30% of cases.

◦ CLINICAL PEARLS ◦

Sinus node dysfunction or disorders of AV conduction are treated with placement of a permanent pacemaker. Treatment of an inducible ventricular arrhythmia entails implantation of an implantable cardioverter defibrillator with or without adjunctive pharmacologic therapy.

Evaluation of Patients Without Structural Heart Disease

In patients without structural heart disease, the most common cause of syncope is neurocardiogenic syncope. Although the mechanism is not completely understood, it appears to involve a neurologic reflex sensitized by states of volume depletion or increased left ventricular contractility. The most common example of this syndrome is the simple vasovagal faint associated with venipuncture. Other typical stimuli include pain, cramping, and emotional stress.

Tilt Table Testing

Head-up tilt table testing is a useful screening tool for neurocardiogenic syncope.

◦ CLINICAL PEARLS ◦

Tilt table testing involves tilting a patient to an 80-degree upright position for 45 minutes under continuous ECG and intermittent blood pressure recording. The upright position causes a redistribution of circulating blood volume to the legs. There is a decrease in cardiac output, followed by a compensatory increase in heart rate and contractility.

In patients susceptible to neurocardiogenic syncope, a reflex vagal response occurs during the test. The sensitivity of the test can be increased with an infusion of isoproterenol, which increases contractility. However, the infusion of isoproterenol also reduces the specificity of the test; therefore, it is important to keep in mind that 5% to 10% of normal control patients will have a positive syncopal response to head-up tilt table testing.

When the etiology of syncope continues to remain elusive, direct recording of the rhythm during syncope can be helpful to exclude a cardiac arrhythmia.

Holter Monitoring

Holter monitors continuously record the cardiac rhythm over a 24-hour (or sometimes 48-hour) period. Holter monitoring may be useful in patients with frequent (daily) episodes of syncope. However, in patients with less frequent episodes, it is less useful. Common findings, such as bradycardia, premature ventricular contractions, and short runs of nonsustained ventricular tachycardia, during Holter monitoring are only relevant if they correlate with the patient's symptoms, which he or she should be recording in a diary. The care provider should be sure to emphasize to the patient the need to record every symptom in the diary (which is issued to the patient along with the Holter monitor) while wearing the monitor.

Loop Event Recorders

Loop event recorders are useful in patients with less frequent episodes of syncope. A loop event recorder is a small, battery-powered device that is worn by the patient and continuously records the patient's ECG. When noteworthy symptoms are experienced, the patient activates the device. On activation, 3 to 4 minutes of prior electrocardiographic activity is stored along with the subsequent 1 to 2 minutes of electrical activity. This recording can be transtelephonically transmitted to a physician for interpretation. The finding of a normal electrical rhythm during a syncopal (or presyncopal) episode excludes a cardiac arrhythmia. Conversely, the finding of a bradyarrhythmia or tachyarrhythmia with syncope can lead to appropriate therapy.

Therapy for Neurocardiogenic Syncope

Excellent pharmacologic therapy is available for patients with neurocardiogenic syncope (Table 2.2). If the symptoms are relatively

TABLE 2.2. *Agents used in the treatment of neurocardiogenic syncope*

Volume-expanding agents
- Salt supplementation
- Fludrocortisone 0.1–0.2 mg q.d.

Beta-adrenergic blocking agents
- Metoprolol 25–50 mg b.i.d.
- Atenolol 25–100 mg q.d.

Selective serotonin reuptake inhibitors
- Fluoxetine 20 mg q.d.
- Paroxetine 10–20 mg q.d.
- Sertraline 50 mg q.d.

Alpha-adrenergic agonist
- Midodrine 5–10 mg t.i.d.

uncommon and the triggers can be identified and avoided, then pharmacologic therapy often is not necessary. Otherwise, the current approach to therapy involves blocking the neurocardiogenic syncope reflex. Volume-expanding agents, such as salt supplementation and fludrocortisone, often are effective, especially in younger patients. Beta-adrenergic blocking agents, such as metoprolol and atenolol, are effective through their negative effects on contractility. The selective serotonin reuptake inhibitors fluoxetine, paroxetine, and sertraline are useful in ameliorating the symptoms at a central level. A recently available alpha-adrenergic agonist, midodrine, causes vasoconstriction, elevates blood pressure, and prevents the neurocardiogenic reflex. This agent also can be used to treat orthostatic hypotension. However, the care provider should administer midodrine with caution, because it can cause marked hypertension.

❍ CLINICAL PEARLS ❍

In young patients with normal hearts, the most common cause of syncope is neurocardiogenic syncope. The prognosis generally is benign.

TABLE 2.3. *Common causes of syncope and their treatments*

Cause	Therapy
Sick sinus syndrome	Permanent pacemaker
Atrioventricular nodal block	Permanent pacemaker
Ventricular tachycardia	Implantable cardioverter defibrillator or pharmacologic therapy
Aortic stenosis	Valve replacement
Neurocardiogenic syncope	Situational avoidance, salt supplementation, pharmacologic agents
Orthostatic hypotension	Discontinuation of offending drug(s), volume repletion, fludrocortisone

SUMMARY

A summary of the common causes of syncope and their treatment is provided in Table 2.3. A complete history and physical examination can identify the etiology of syncope in approximately 50% of cases. When the etiology remains uncertain, it is critical to rule out cardiovascular causes, because the associated mortality is high. Patients with evidence of structural heart disease or an abnormal ECG should be hospitalized and referred for electrophysiologic testing. In younger patients with structurally normal hearts, syncope usually has a benign prognosis. Head-up tilt table testing can help identify neurocardiogenic syncope. When the cause still remains elusive, event recorder monitoring may be the best way to exclude a significant arrhythmia.

3

Atrial Fibrillation

Alvin Blaustein and *Jaggarao S. Nattama

Baylor College of Medicine, Non-invasive Laboratory,
*Electrophysiology and Pacing, Houston V. A. Medical Center,
Houston, Texas 77030

Atrial fibrillation is the most common arrhythmia requiring treatment. Atrial fibrillation rarely occurs as a primary arrhythmia; rather, it usually occurs in the setting of organic heart diseases. During atrial fibrillation, there is no organized contraction of the atria. A substantial component of the morbidity associated with atrial fibrillation, and a strong impetus for treatment, is that during atrial fibrillation there is relative stasis of blood in the left atrium, particularly in the left atrial appendage. In this setting, a thrombus may form and later embolize to the cerebral circulation, resulting in stroke. The loss of organized atrial contraction may decrease effective filling of the ventricles during diastole, which in turn may decrease cardiac output and lead to pulmonary edema. Finally, the fast ventricular response rate in some patients with atrial fibrillation may lead to cardiac symptoms and morbidity.

For these reasons, a number of important clinical trials have been performed that now allow practitioners to make more informed decisions regarding the management of atrial fibrillation (although some other issues regarding management remain unresolved). In this chapter, the management of the patient with atrial fibrillation is discussed and algorithms regarding the care of patients are presented.

DIAGNOSIS

History

The majority of patients who develop atrial fibrillation either have few symptoms or are asymptomatic. Thus, the onset of atrial fibrillation often is unrecognized. Symptoms that may suggest onset of atrial fibrillation include palpitations, fast and/or irregular heart beat, decreased exercise

21

tolerance, fatigue, and symptoms associated with pulmonary congestion or low cardiac output.

Physical Examination

The primary finding on physical examination suggestive of atrial fibrillation is an often rapid, grossly irregular pulse. One also may note a varying in intensity of the first heart sound.

Electrocardiogram

The definitive diagnosis of atrial fibrillation is the finding of irregularly irregular QRS complexes and the absence of any evidence of organized atrial activity (either P waves or flutter waves) on the electrocardiogram.

◆ CLINICAL PEARLS ◆

Both multifocal atrial tachycardia and atrial flutter may produce irregularly irregular QRS complexes. However, with multifocal atrial tachycardia, P waves of differing morphology precede the QRS complexes. With atrial flutter, flutter waves often are visible between the QRS complexes.

OVERALL APPROACH TO THE PATIENT WITH ATRIAL FIBRILLATION

The first step in the management of patients discovered to have atrial fibrillation is deciding if the patient needs to be promptly hospitalized. After this initial step, the next three steps are to (i) control the ventricular response rate, (ii) prevent thromboembolism, and (iii) convert the patient back to normal sinus rhythm. This approach is illustrated in Fig. 3.1. *Proper management will reduce the likelihood of death and disability due to stroke and heart failure resulting from persistent tachycardia.* In addition, possible direct or contributing causes to the development of atrial fibrillation should be considered and investigated.

DECIDING WHICH PATIENTS NEED HOSPITALIZATION

Factors that should lead to prompt hospitalization are summarized in Table 3.1. The decision as to which patients seen in the outpatient setting require prompt hospitalization and treatment is based primarily on an assessment of the patients' hemodynamic status and symptoms.

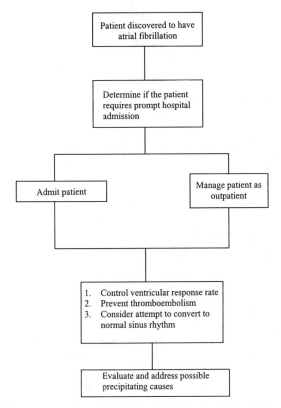

FIG. 3.1. Overall approach to the patient with atrial fibrillation.

Physical Examination

Blood pressure should be assessed carefully to see if the patient is hypotensive. The examination should look for findings suggestive of congestive heart failure (particularly pulmonary edema as well as the presence of a third heart sound [S3]) and those that suggest structural heart disease (including murmurs suggestive of mitral stenosis, aortic stenosis, or hypertrophic cardiomyopathy).

TABLE 3.1. *Indications for prompt hospital admission*

- Rapid ventricular response rate (>160 beats/min)
- Congestive heart failure
- Angina
- Hypotension
- Presence of significant organic heart disease

❖ CLINICAL PEARLS ❖

Because not all ventricular contractions lead to a significant ejection of blood from the left ventricle in patients with atrial fibrillation and rapid ventricular response rates, counting the number of palpable peripheral pulsations over a certain duration of time to calculate the ventricular response rate may underestimate the actual ventricular response rate. Thus, the ventricular response rate is best determined by inspection of the electrocardiogram (ECG).

History

Patients should be questioned regarding symptoms associated with congestive heart failure (dyspnea on exertion, orthopnea. and paroxysmal nocturnal dyspnea) and whether they have had or are having symptoms associated with cardiac ischemia and angina.

Electrocardiogram

Because patients with rapid ventricular response rates should be considered for prompt treatment and hospitalization, the ECG should be used to determine the ventricular response rate. Patients with ECG evidence of prior myocardial infarction, left ventricular hypertrophy, or ongoing ischemia should be treated more aggressively, as these findings are associated with a greater incidence of atrial fibrillation-associated adverse events.

CONTROLLING THE VENTRICULAR RESPONSE RATE

Patients with rapid ventricular response rates (greater than 150 to 160 beats/ min), particularly if they are symptomatic, may require more urgent treatment to slow the response rate. In such patients, intravenous administration of atrioventricular (AV) nodal blocking agents is used. In more stable patients in whom the need to slow the ventricular response rate is less pressing, initial and maintenance therapy with oral agents is acceptable.

❖ CLINICAL PEARLS ❖

Patients with atrial fibrillation and rapid ventricular response rates who are unstable (florid congestive heart failure, severe angina, hypotension) should be treated with prompt synchronized cardioversion.

Intravenous Agents

The use of intravenous agents to slow the ventricular response rate should only be performed in a monitored setting. Intravenous beta blocker or calcium channel blocker preparations are the usual first-line agents. The negative inotropic effects of these agents must be weighed against the need to rapidly decrease the heart rate in patients, particularly those in congestive heart failure. Intravenous digoxin is not suited for *urgent* rate control, because onset of its effects is delayed for 1 hour and its maximal effects do not occur until approximately 3 hours after administration. Suggested dosing schedules for intravenous agents that slow the ventricular response rate are given in Table 3.2.

TABLE 3.2. *Selected intravenous agents and possible treatment regimens used to slow the ventricular response rate in patients with atrial fibrillation*

Medication	Intravenous loading dose	Usual subsequent i.v. or oral maintenance dose
Beta blockers		
Metoprolol (Lopressor)	• 5 mg i.v. q5min as tolerated and necessary	• 50–100 mg p.o. b.i.d.
Esmolol	• 500 µg/kg[a] over 1 min; then 50 µg/kg/min[a] for 4 min • May repeat loading dose and increase maintenance dose by 50 µg/kg/min[a] q5min as tolerated and necessary	• Continuous i.v. infusion of 150–200 µg/kg/min
Calcium channel blockers		
Diltiazem (Cardizem)	• Initial 0.25 mg/kg over 2 min • After 15 min, if necessary, can give additional 0.35 mg/kg over 2 min as tolerated and necessary	• Continuous i.v. infusion of 5–15 mg/h i.v. • 30–120 mg p.o. t.i.d. 120–369 mg SR q.d.
Verapamil	• 2.5–5 mg i.v. over 2–3 min • May repeat dose if tolerated and as necessary	• 40–120 mg p.o. t.i.d. or 180–360 mg SR q.d.
Cardiac glycosides		
Digoxin	• Initial 0.25–0.5 mg i.v. bolus • Subsequent doses of 0.25 mg i.v. q6–8h until rate control or total dose of 1.0–1.5 mg given then	0.125–0.37 mg p.o. q.d.

[a] Note dose is in *micro*grams, not milligrams.

Oral Agents

Beta blockers, calcium channel blockers, and digoxin are all acceptable oral agents for controlling the ventricular response rate. In general, beta blockers and calcium channel blockers provide better ventricular rate control than digoxin, particularly during periods of exertion or exercise.

Beta blockers are preferred in those with coronary artery disease, given their antiischemic and cardioprotective properties. Beta blockers should be used with caution in patients with depressed left ventricular ejection fraction (less than 40%) and avoided in those with ongoing congestive heart failure. Calcium channel blockers may be desirable in those who are hypertensive. Calcium channel blockers generally should not be used in those with depressed ejection fractions. Digoxin may be desirable in those with depressed ejection fractions and congestive heart failure, given its modest positive inotropic actions. If one agent alone fails to adequately control ventricular response rate, a second class of agents can be utilized in conjunction with the initial agent. Suggested dosing schedules for oral agents that slow the ventricular response rate are given in Table 3.3.

◄► CLINICAL PEARLS ◄►

In patients who present with ventricular rates less than 110, use AV nodal blocking medications cautiously. Slow responses in the absence of rate-reducing medications indicate disease of the cardiac conducting system.

PREVENTING THROMBOEMBOLISM WITH WARFARIN

The greatest concern in patients with atrial fibrillation is that thrombus will form in the left atrium and subsequently embolize to the cerebral circulation, causing a stroke. There are two means of preventing thromboembolism: (i) restoring sinus rhythm and (ii) long-term anticoagulation with warfarin (Coumadin).

In most patients, it is desirable to chemically or electrically cardiovert the patient to restore normal sinus rhythm. Some patients, however, will prove refractory to cardioversion or will repeatedly revert to atrial fibrillation. Patients with persistent or recurrent atrial fibrillation should be considered for chronic anticoagulation, as discussed in the following section.

Who to Treat with Long-term Anticoagulation

Several factors have been identified that are associated with an increased risk of thromboembolism and stroke in patients with atrial fibrillation. The presence of one or more of these factors increases the impetus to

TABLE 3.3. *Selected treatment regimens for oral agents and possible treatment regimens used to slow and control the ventricular response rate in patients with atrial fibrillation*

Medication	Initial dose	Usual maintenance dose
Beta blockers		
Atenolol (Tenormin)	• 50 mg p.o. q.d.	• 50–200 mg p.o. q.d.
Metoprolol (Lopressor)	• 50 mg p.o. b.i.d. regular duration acting meto-prolol	• 50–100 mg p.o. b.i.d. regular duration acting metoprolol • 100–200 mg p.o. b.i.d. long-acting Toprol XL
Calcium channel blockers		
Diltiazem (Cardizem)	• 30 mg p.o. t.i.d.–q.i.d. regular duration acting diltiazem	• 30–90 mg p.o. t.i.d.–q.i.d. regular duration acting diltiazem • 60–180 mg p.o. b.i.d. longer-acting Cardizem SR • 180–300 mg p.o. long-acting Cardizem CD • 120–360 mg p.o. long-acting Dilacor XR • 120–360 mg p.o. long-acting Tiazac
Verapamil	• 40 mg p.o. t.i.d. regular duration acting verapamil	• 120–240 mg p.o. q.d.–b.i.d. long-acting Calan SR or Isoptin ST • 120–480 mg p.o. long-acting Veralin
Cardiac glycosides		
Digoxin	• 1.0–1.5 mg p.o. given in divided doses over 1–3 days	• 0.125–0.375 mg p.o. q.d.

anticoagulate patients with warfarin. These factors are listed in Table 3.4. Patients with any of these risk factors should receive warfarin unless the risk of bleeding is prohibitive or unless sinus rhythm can be restored permanently.

⟴ CLINICAL PEARLS ⟴

Patients who have intermittent or "paroxysmal" atrial fibrillation are at as much risk for stroke as those with chronic (continuous) atrial fibrillation and should similarly be considered for long-term anticoagulation therapy.

Patients without any of these clinical or echocardiographic risk factors are said to have "lone" atrial fibrillation, and the yearly risk of stroke

TABLE 3.4. *Factors associated with an increased risk of thromboembolism and stroke in patients with atrial fibrillation*

- Hypertension
- Diabetes
- Age >75 years
- Left ventricular ejection fraction <40%
- Congestive heart failure
- Structural heart disease
- Stroke, transient ischemic attack, or systemic embolism

is much lower (less than 1% in some populations). Although anticoagulation still is effective in preventing stroke, the magnitude of benefit is not as great. In patients with lone atrial fibrillation who are less than 65 years old, aspirin therapy is generally considered adequate. These patients should be switched to warfarin therapy if they develop any of the risk factors associated with an increased risk of stroke. In patients 65 years of age or older, warfarin therapy is recommended. In such older patients who cannot be treated with warfarin, aspirin 325 mg q.d. may somewhat reduce the risk of stroke.

Treatment with Warfarin

Warfarin therapy may be initiated in either the inpatient or outpatient setting. Patients should not be "loaded" with warfarin but rather begun on a dose estimated to be what will be required for long-term maintenance. Usual maintenance doses range from 2.5 to 5 mg p.o. q.d. Warfarin doses should be adjusted to maintain the international normalized ratio (INR) between 2.0 and 3.0. The INR should be checked initially weekly or biweekly until a therapeutic regimen is determined, and then it should be checked monthly.

Medications and Foods that Interact with Warfarin and Anticoagulation

Many medications and some foods can either directly interact with warfarin or can act on the body's anticoagulation system to either increase or decrease INR levels. Because of this, it is worthwhile to acquaint patients with these medications and foods. Because it is impossible for either the primary care provider or the patient to memorize such a list, one is provided in the chapter on anticoagulation (see Chapter 10). You may wish to photocopy this table and give it to each patient.

Interrupting Warfarin Therapy

If warfarin must be interrupted for a procedure (elective surgery, dental procedures, biopsies, etc.), there are two possible management strategies. One strategy is to stop warfarin therapy 3 to 4 days before the procedure and admit the patient to the hospital for anticoagulation with intravenous heparin therapy until the procedure. Use this strategy for patients at higher risk of thromboembolic disease (Table 3.4). The second strategy is to stop warfarin therapy 3 to 4 days before the procedure and not anticoagulate the patient with heparin in the days before the procedure.

With either strategy, warfarin therapy should be restarted after the procedure. Patients at higher risk of thromboembolism should be anticoagulated with heparin until the INR has reached a therapeutic level.

RESTORING NORMAL SINUS RHYTHM

Cardioversion to sinus rhythm may be accomplished either pharmacologically or through electrical cardioversion. The timing of cardioversion depends predominantly on whether the patient is stable or unstable, and how long the patient has been in atrial fibrillation. Three possible protocols for converting patients are discussed at the end of this section and are summarized in Table 3.5. An algorithm for deciding on which protocol to choose is presented in Fig. 3.2.

TABLE 3.5. *Protocols for cardioverting and managing patients with atrial fibrillation*

Protocol	Anticoagulation regimen cardioversion	Need for TEE prior to cardioversion	Cardioversion method	Need for post-cardioversion antiarrhythmic therapy
Protocol 1: Early cardioversion with AF duration <48 h	• Start heparin and warfarin therapy prior to cardioversion • Continue warfarin for 1 month after cardioversion	• Not necessary if no history of prior embolism	• Intravenous pharmacologic agent if heart structurally normal • Electrical if known structural heart disease	• Not necessary if structurally normal heart • Recommended for 6–12 mo if structural and/or organic heart disease
Protocol 2: Early cardioversion with AF duration either unknown or >48 h	• Start heparin and warfarin prior to cardioversion • Continue warfarin for 1 month after cardioversion	Needed prior to cardioversion: • If no clot, then cardiovert • If clot detected, then go to protocol 3	• Electrical cardioversion preferred, especially if patient has known heart disease	• Recommended for 12 mo
Protocol 3: Delayed cardioversion	• Warfarin for 3–4 wk prior to conversion • Continue warfarin for 1 month after cardioversion	• Not necessary if no history of prior embolism	• Electrical cardioversion preferred	• Recommended for 12 mo

AF, atrial fibrillation; TEE, transesophageal echocardiography.

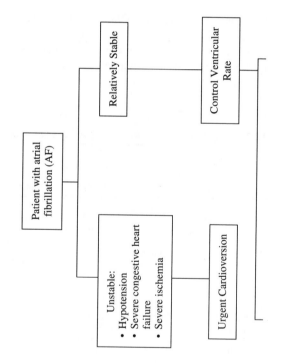

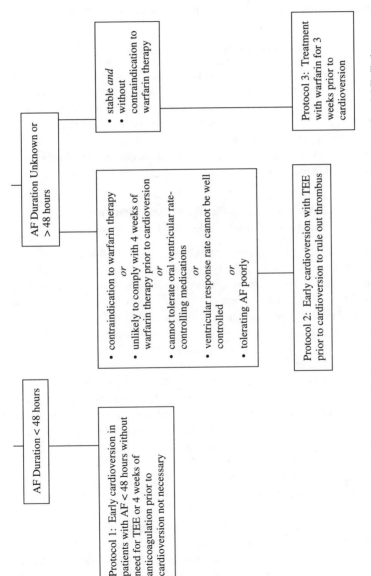

FIG. 3.2. Algorithm for choosing the approach to cardioverting patients with atrial fibrillation.

Which Patients Should Be Considered for Cardioversion

Because there are multiple benefits to restoring normal sinus rhythm, particularly decreasing the risk of stroke, an attempt at cardioversion should be considered in all patients. Patients with depressed ejection fractions, congestive heart failure, and contraindications to long-term warfarin therapy are likely to benefit most from cardioversion.

Which Patients Require Urgent Cardioversion

Patients who are unstable (hypotension, pulmonary edema, severe ischemia) should be considered for urgent cardioversion. Although there may be some small risk of stroke with cardioversion, in unstable patients the benefits of restoring sinus rhythm generally outweigh the small risk of stroke. If possible, reversing acidosis, hypoxemia, or other metabolic disturbances and slowing AV conduction improve the likelihood of successful cardioversion.

Protocol 1: Early Cardioversion in Patients with Duration of Atrial Fibrillation Less than 48 Hours

Patients in whom the onset of atrial fibrillation occurred less than 48 hours prior to presentation have a very low risk of systemic embolization with cardioversion. Begin anticoagulation with intravenous heparin at once (at the time of this writing, there are no data to support the use of low-molecular-weight heparins) and arrange for cardioversion within 24 hours. Oral anticoagulation therapy should also be started at this time, because it will be continued for 4 weeks in patients successfully cardioverted and indefinitely in patients in whom cardioversion is unsuccessful.

Synchronized electrical shock successfully converts 90% of patients with atrial fibrillation. Intravenous medications are less effective, but they have their best success in patients when the duration of atrial fibrillation is short and in patients with little or no structural and/or organic heart disease. Protocols for cardioverting patients are given in Table 3.5, and several intravenous agents currently utilized in the chemical cardioversion of atrial fibrillation are listed in Table 3.6. A checklist and protocol for electrical cardioversion is discussed in the following and are given in Table 3.7.

After cardioversion, patients with structural and/or organic heart disease should receive antiarrhythmic therapy for at least 12 months to sustain the patient in normal sinus rhythm. Patients with structurally normal hearts and no history of prior atrial fibrillation episodes can be observed without initiating long-term antiarrhythmic therapy.

TABLE 3.6. *Several intravenously administered pharmacologic agents used in converting atrial fibrillation to normal sinus rhythm and possible dosing protocols*

Agent	Initial dose	Subsequent treatment	Comments
Ibutilide	1 mg i.v. over 10 min, may repeat after 20 min	• Need long-term oral therapy with different agent	• Continuous monitoring for prolonged QT (QT_c >450 ms) and arrhythmia • Watch for QT prolongation and torsades de pointes
Procainamide	50 mg/min i.v. to total dose of 10–14 mg/kg (usually 1 g total)	• Procaine SR 500–1,000mg p.o. q6h • Procanbid 1,000–2,000 mg p.o. q12 h	• Continuous monitoring for prolonged QT (QT_c >450 ms), arrhythmia, and hypotension • Watch for QT prolongation and torsades de pointes

Note that all antiarrhythmics have serious and potentially life-threatening side effects and one should consult the manufacturer's monogram and thoroughly familiarize oneself with all the precautions, cautions, and contraindications of the medication before use.

As noted earlier, in patients who are successfully cardioverted, warfarin therapy should still be prescribed for 4 weeks, because with cardioversion there may be "atrial stunning" and the patient may still be at risk for thrombus formation for 2 to 3 weeks.

Protocol 2: Early Cardioversion in Patients with Duration of Atrial Fibrillation Either Unknown or Less Than 48 Hours

In many patients, the primary care provider does not know the duration of atrial fibrillation. In these patients, it must be presumed that the patient has been in atrial fibrillation long enough (more than 48 hours) that there is a risk that thrombus has formed in the left atrium.

In some patients, it is desirable to perform early cardioversion rather than anticoagulate the patient 4 weeks prior to cardioversion (as discussed in protocol 3). Consider patients with the following indications for early cardioversion:

• Contraindications to warfarin therapy
• Cannot comply with warfarin therapy
• Will not tolerate oral ventricular rate controlling medications
• Ventricular response rates cannot be well controlled
• Tolerating the atrial fibrillation poorly.

TABLE 3.7. *Steps in the preparation for and electrical cardioversion of the patient with atrial fibrillation*

- Patient should be NPO for >6 h
- Ensure that potassium, magnesium, digoxin, partial thromboplastin time, and/or international normalized ratio levels are normal or therapeutic
- Ensure that signed informed consent has been obtained
- Have anesthesia present to administer sedation and monitor the patient's airway
- Cover the paddles completely with conductive gel or use conductive adhesive patches
- Check that on the defibrillator "synchronized cardioversion" is selected and that the monitor shows that the machine is tracking the QRS complexes
- Place paddles in correct positions; apply firm pressure
- Choose an initial discharge of 100 J; if unsuccessful increase sequentially to 200, 300, and then 360 J. Fewer than 5% require >200 J.

To evaluate the risk of embolism in the period after cardioversion, perform a transesophageal echocardiogram. In the absence of intracardiac clot in the left atrial appendage, the risk of embolism is very low.

In patients who are to be managed in this manner, begin heparin and warfarin therapy and discuss the case with a cardiologist who performs transesophageal echocardiograms. If no thrombus is detected, it generally is safe to proceed with cardioversion within the next 24 hours. After cardioversion, patients should be maintained on warfarin for 1 month at an INR of approximately 2.5 to 3.5 and antiarrhythmic therapy for 12 months (or longer in the presence of significant organic heart disease).

Protocol 3: Delayed Cardioversion

Many stable patients with atrial fibrillation can be managed with a strategy of placing them on warfarin for 3 to 4 weeks and then converting the rhythm. Anticoagulation should be maintained at an INR of 2.5 to 3.5 during this period, because the patient is being treated as though a thrombus is present in the atrium. Patients who fall below the therapeutic range for any substantial time may not obtain the maximum protection. Those who should be considered for this strategy include:

- Patients with prior embolic stroke
- Patients in whom a transesophageal echocardiogram is contraindicated or prefer not to undergo one
- Those who on transesophageal echocardiography are found to have an atrial thrombus.

After cardioversion, patients should be continued on warfarin for 1 month, because with cardioversion there may be "atrial stunning" and the patient may still be at risk for thrombus formation for several weeks. Antiarrhythmic therapy should continue for at least 12 months or longer if there is significant organic and/or structural heart disease.

METHODS OF CARDIOVERSION

Either medications or synchronized electrical shock can convert patients to sinus rhythm. Stable patients should be triaged and treated as outlined in the three protocols before attempting cardioversion.

Pharmacologic Cardioversion

Pharmacologic attempts at cardioversion are most likely to be successful in patients with atrial fibrillation of short duration and/or structurally normal (or nearly normal) hearts. Agents that have been utilized to convert atrial fibrillation include ibutilide (Corvert), procainamide, quinidine, propafenone (Rhythmol), and sotalol (Betapace).

Ibutilide (Corvert) is approved for the conversion of recent-onset (less than 90 days) atrial fibrillation. The usual dosage of ibutilide is 1 mg given intravenously over 10 minutes. If the arrhythmia does not terminate within 10 minutes after the end of the infusion, a second 10-minute intravenous infusion of 1 mg may be administered. *Patients treated with ibutilide and other antiarrhythmic agents that prolong the QT interval should undergo continuous telemetry monitoring to follow for QT-segment prolongation and the development of torsades de pointes.*

Electrical Cardioversion

Synchronized direct-current shock converts 90% of patients (although fewer than 50% who are untreated with subsequent antiarrhythmic therapy will remain in sinus rhythm). *Note that only practitioners knowledgeable and experienced in Advanced Cardiac Life Support (ACLS) procedures and electrical cardioversion and defibrillation should attempt electrical cardioversion.*

MAINTAINING SINUS RHYTHM

Regardless of how sinus rhythm is restored, fewer than 40% of those cardioverted will sustain sinus rhythm 1 year later without adjunctive therapy. Medications that have been utilized to sustain normal sinus rhythm include amiodarone (Cordarone), procainamide, quinidine, and sotalol (Betapace). Quinidine or procainamide increases the likelihood of remaining in sinus rhythm to approximately 50% to 55%. Quinidine

Table 3.8 *Selected pharmacologic agents for maintaining normal sinus rhythm in patients converted from atrial fibrillation*

Medication	Dose
Amiodarone	200 mg b.i.d.–t.i.d. for 1–3 weeks then 200 mg q.d.–b.i.d.
Procaine SR Procanbid	• 500–1000 mg p.o. q6h of Procaine SR • 1000–2000 mg p.o. q12h of Procanbid
Propafenone	125–225 mg q8h or 300 mg q12h
Quinidine gluconate	324–648 mg p.o. q8h
Sotalol	120 mg p.o. t.i.d.
Azimilide (Stedicor)	100–125 mg p.o. b.i.d. × 3 days then 100–125 mg p.o. q.d.
Dofetilide (Tikosyn)	250–500 micrograms p.o. b.i.d

should not be utilized in patients with depressed left ventricular ejection fraction. Newer medications, particularly amiodarone, may be more effective in maintaining sinus rhythm (70% to 75% sinus rhythm after 1 year). Several other new promising agents (currently in the final testing and approval stages at the time of this writing), including azimilide (Stedicor) and dofetilide (Tikosyn), appear to be useful in maintaining sinus rhythm.

Monitoring During the Loading Period

During early dosing of these agents, patients should undergo continuous telemetry monitoring and daily 12-lead ECGs to assure that the QT interval does not become prolonged, that the patient does not develop bradycardia or heart block, and that the patient does not develop the lethal ventricular arrhythmia torsades de pointes. Amiodarone has the

Table 3.8 *Continued*

Major side effects	Comments
• Bradycardia and AV node block • CNS effects (particularly ataxia) • Pulmonary fibrosis • Hypothyroidism and hyperthyroidism • LFT elevations • Photosensitivity	• Monitor for bradycardia, heart block, severe QT prolongation during loading phase • Follow CXR, TSH, and LFTs every 6 months while on therapy • Can significantly raise digoxin level and increase INR—decrease doses of digoxin and warfarin
• QT prolongation and torsades de pointes • Lupus-like syndrome	• Monitor for QT prolongation and torsades de pointes • Monitor CBC; watch for symptoms of SLE
• Torsades de pointes • Beta-blocking properties related side effects (worsening of CHF, etc.)	• Monitor for QRS interval prolongation and torsades de pointes
• QT prolongation and torsades de pointes • Diarrhea	• Monitor for QT prolongation and torsades de pointes • Do not use in patients with depressed ejection fractions • Markedly raises digoxin level—decrease digoxin dose
• QT prolongation and torsades de pointes • Beta-blocking properties related side effects (worsening of CHF, etc.)	• Monitor for QT prolongation and torsades de pointes
• QT prolongation and torsades de pointes	• Monitor for QT prolongation and torsades de pointes
• QT prolongation and torsades de pointes	• Monitor for QT prolongation and torsades de pointes

All antiarrhythmics have serious and potentially life-threatening side effects and one should consult the manufacturer's monogram and thoroughly familiarize oneself with all the precautions, cautions, and contraindications of the medication before use. Although commonly used in the treatment of normal sinus rhythm, listed drugs may not be approved by the Food and Drug Administration for this use.

CBC, complete blood count; CHF, congestive heart failure; CNS, central nervous system; CXR, chest x-ray; LFT, liver function test; SLE, systemic lupus erythematosis; TSH, thyroid-stimulating hormone.

advantage of little, if any, proarrhythmic properties and, particularly when compared to some other antiarrhythmic agents, is relatively safe to use in patients with depressed left ventricular ejection fraction. Newer agents, such as azimilide, may not require in-hospital telemetry monitoring during the loading period. Several agents that are utilized in the maintenance of normal sinus rhythm are listed in Table 3.8. *Note that, as with utilizing the intravenous agents, all antiarrhythmics have serious and potentially life-threatening side effects; therefore, one should consult*

TABLE 3.9. *Possible direct and contributing causes to the development of atrial fibrillation*

- Dilated or diseased atria
- Sinoatrial node disease ("sick sinus syndrome")
- Valvular heart disease
- Coronary artery disease
- Hypertension
- Advanced age
- Metabolic disturbances or toxins (particularly ETOH)
- Pericardial disease (pericarditis, etc.)
- Pulmonary embolus
- Thyrotoxicosis

the manufacturer's monogram and thoroughly familiarize oneself with all the precautions, cautions, and contraindications of the medication before use. Note also that although commonly used in the treatment and maintenance of normal sinus rhythm, not all listed drugs are approved by the Food and Drug Administration for these uses.

INVESTIGATING THE CAUSE OF ATRIAL FIBRILLATION

Direct and contributing causes to the development of atrial fibrillation are listed in Table 3.9. Not every patient needs to be evaluated for every possible cause of atrial fibrillation. The patients' history, physical examination, and ECG should be used to help guide the evaluation. Cardiac echocardiography frequently is obtained, as it is useful not only in assessing for a dilated left atrium or depressed ejection fraction, but it also can determine whether the patient has any type of structural heart disease, which will help guide initial therapy and long-term management.

SUMMARY

Morbidity associated with atrial fibrillation includes stroke and congestive heart failure. Steps involved in the care of patients with atrial fibrillation include determining if the patient needs prompt hospitalization, controlling the ventricular response rate, preventing thromboembolism, and considering an attempt at converting the patient back to normal sinus rhythm. Precipitating causes should be considered and addressed as indicated.

4

Evaluation and Management of Patients with Valvular Heart Disease

Sherif F. Nagueh

Baylor College of Medicine, Section of Cardiology,
Methodist Hospital, Houston, Texas 77030

Valvular heart disease affects nearly 5 million Americans. The appropriate recognition and management of valvular heart disease frequently will lead to a normal lifespan, whereas the misdiagnosis and/or mismanagement of valvular heart disease will result in the development of intractable heart failure and a shortened lifespan. Recent advances in noninvasive imaging modalities have allowed better evaluation and understanding of the pathophysiology and natural history of valvular heart disease. In this chapter, the diagnosis and management of patients with mitral regurgitation (MR), aortic stenosis (AS), and aortic regurgitation (AR) will be discussed. The evaluation of other, less common valvular lesions is beyond the intended scope of this chapter.

MITRAL REGURGITATION

Mitral regurgitation results from a disruption of the mitral valve apparatus, which consists of the mitral valve annulus, the mitral leaflets, the chordae tendineae, and the papillary muscles. When abnormalities of any of these four components cause blood to regurgitate backward from the left ventricle (LV) into the left atrium, the regurgitation is classified as *primary*. When disease states (e.g., heart failure) cause ventricular dilation with resultant misalignment of the papillary muscles, the regurgitation is considered to be *secondary*.

Mitral regurgitation may develop acutely (acute MR) over a matter of minutes, or the lesion may develop insidiously over a period of decades (chronic MR). Given that the primary care provider is more likely to

TABLE 4.1. *Causes of mitral regurgitation*

Mitral valve prolapse
Ischemic heart disease with papillary muscle dysfunction
Infective endocarditis
Rheumatic fever
Congenital
Drugs (ergot alkaloids, anorectic drugs)
Marfan syndrome
Systemic lupus erythematosis
Hypertrophic cardiomyopathy
Trauma (ruptured chordae tendineae)

encounter patients with chronic MR than acute MR, the major focus of this section will be chronic MR. The most common etiologies for chronic MR are listed in Table 4.1. As shown, mitral valve prolapse is probably the most common cause of MR in North America, followed by ischemic heart disease. Other relatively common causes include infective endocarditis, systemic lupus erythematosis, and certain drugs (ergot alkaloids, anorectic drugs). Mitral regurgitation not only leads to an increase in left atrial pressure, but it also places a volume overload on the LV. As the disease becomes more chronic, both left atrial and left ventricular dilation will occur. The increased volume of the left atrium and LV allows the regurgitant volume to be accommodated at lower left ventricular end-diastolic pressures, thus reducing the symptoms of pulmonary congestion. This compensated stage may persist for several years. If uncorrected, it eventually leads to left ventricular dysfunction and heart failure. In patients with MR, a decrease in ejection fraction usually indicates the presence of muscle dysfunction.

✪ CLINICAL PEARLS ✪

Ejection fraction usually is increased (i.e., greater than 60% to 65%) in MR, because blood is simultaneously ejected into the left atrium as well as into the aorta. Thus, the observation that a patient with MR has "only" a "normal" ejection fraction of 50% to 55% generally indicates the presence of left ventricular dysfunction that requires evaluation for valve repair/replacement.

DIAGNOSIS OF MITRAL REGURGITATION

Symptoms

Valuable clues regarding the etiology of MR may be elicited from the history. For example, a history of angina and/or myocardial infarction suggests an ischemic etiology. A history of sharp atypical chest pain, particularly in an asthenic woman, raises the possibility of mitral valve prolapse. Patients may relate a prior history of rheumatic fever as a child, infectious endocarditis, or ingestion of ergotamine or diet pills. In general, patients with chronic MR frequently are asymptomatic for a period of years before left ventricular dysfunction ensues. The onset of left ventricular dysfunction is heralded by a change in the patient's functional capacity or symptoms referable to the onset of heart failure (shortness of breath, paroxysmal dyspnea, and orthopnea).

Physical Examination

The left ventricular apex in chronic MR is displaced laterally and downward. The typical murmur of MR is a holosystolic apical murmur that radiates to the axilla. This murmur often is accompanied by a thrill. A mitral valve click may be heard in patients with mitral valve prolapse at mid to late systole. These clicks usually are followed by a late systolic murmur. Maneuvers that decrease the left ventricular end diastolic volume (standing and Valsalva) will result in an earlier onset of the click and a longer duration of the murmur. Alternatively, increasing left ventricular volume (for example, being in supine position) will result in a later onset of the click and a shorter duration of the murmur. Patients with rheumatic heart disease may have additional findings, such as an opening snap and aortic murmurs.

Electrocardiographic Findings

There are no diagnostic findings on the electrocardiogram (ECG) that are specific for MR. Commonly, however, the ECG will disclose signs of left atrial enlargement, left ventricular hypertrophy, and/or atrial arrhythmias.

Chest X-ray Findings

There are no diagnostic findings on the chest X-ray film that are specific for MR. Findings that are observed with significant chronic MR include cardiomegaly, left atrial enlargement, and/or pulmonary venous congestion.

Noninvasive Findings

Echocardiography is essential in the assessment of MR. During echocardiography, left ventricular dimension and LV can be assessed, as well as the etiology of MR (redundant thick mitral leaflets indicative of prolapse, or rheumatic, etc). Color flow Doppler provides an estimate of the severity of MR. If other valvular lesions are present, their hemodynamic significance can be readily ascertained. Pulmonary artery systolic pressure can be calculated from the Doppler as well. A transesophageal echocardiogram should be obtained in most patients with nonrheumatic MR to determine whether the mitral valve can be repaired.

✧ CLINICAL PEARLS ✧

Color flow Doppler may significantly underestimate or overestimate the amount of regurgitation depending on the echocardiographic imaging plane that is used, as well as the patient's volume status and blood pressure at the time of the study. Therefore, it is useful in assessing the severity of chronic MR to remember that significant chronic MR almost always will be accompanied by a significant increase in left ventricular end-diastolic dimension (greater than 55 mm).

Invasive Studies

Most patients who require mitral valve surgery generally will be of the age where they may have coexisting coronary artery disease. Prior to any planned mitral valve surgery, patients generally should undergo a diagnostic cardiac catheterization. Occasionally, there will be a discrepancy between the clinical and the noninvasive assessment of the severity of MR, in which case a cardiac catheterization may help to resolve the discrepant findings. In addition to coronary angiography, cardiac catheterization will determine the size and function of the LV as well as the severity of MR (the latter only semiquantitatively). Right heart catheterization is needed for the determination of left atrial and pulmonary artery pressures.

MANAGEMENT OF CHRONIC MITRAL REGURGITATION

Surgical Therapy

The only definitive treatment for MR is mitral valve surgery. The timing of mitral valve surgery should, ideally, occur before irreversible left ventricular dysfunction has developed. To achieve a surgical outcome that allows for a normal postoperative lifespan, relief of symptoms, and normal postoperative ejection performance, MR should be corrected before left ventricular ejection fraction falls below 60%, or before echocardiographic end-systolic dimensions exceed 45 mm. Further delay in operation may result in persistent postoperative left ventricular dysfunction and/or a reduced lifespan. Other indications for referring a patient for surgery (Table 4.2) include (i) symptomatic patients with normal left ventricular size (left ventricular end-diastolic dimension less than 45 mm)

TABLE 4.2. *Guidelines for referral for valve replacement in mitral regurgitation*

Symptoms	ESD (mm)		EF	Course of action
None	<45		>0.60	Observe
Mild	<45		>0.60	Observe
>Mild	<45		>0.60	Refer for further evaluation
None	>45	or	<0.60	Refer for further evaluation
Yes	>45	or	<0.60	Refer for further evaluation

EF, ejection fraction; ESD, end-systolic dimension.
(Adapted from Carabello BA. Recognition and management of patients with valvular heart disease. In Goldman L, Braunwald E, eds. *Primary cardiology,* 1st ed. Philadelphia: WB Saunders, 1998:381.)

and function (ejection fraction greater than 60%); (ii) asymptomatic patients with a left ventricular end-systolic dimension greater than 45 mm and an ejection fraction less than 60%; and (3) symptomatic patients with a left ventricular end-systolic dimension greater than 45 mm and an ejection fraction less than 60%.

Currently, three types of operation are performed for the correction of MR: mitral valve replacement with removal of the mitral valve apparatus, mitral valve replacement with preservation of at least part of the mitral valve apparatus, and mitral valve repair in which a prosthetic valve is avoided and the native valve is reconstructed so that it becomes competent. Mitral valve repair offers two advantages: first, it preserves the mitral valve apparatus and therefore leads to less postoperative left ventricular dysfunction; and second, it offers freedom from anticoagulants for patients in sinus rhythm. Accordingly, mitral valve repair is the preferred approach whenever possible.

Medical Therapy

Medical therapy in MR is reserved for acute symptomatic MR (see following) and for patients with chronic symptomatic MR deemed not to be surgical candidates. Unlike in AR, where the use of vasodilators may forestall surgery in patients with asymptomatic chronic disease (see following), there is no convincing evidence that vasodilator therapy is of benefit in chronic asymptomatic MR. In patients with symptomatic chronic MR that is inoperable, digoxin, diuretics, and vasodilators form the mainstay of medical therapy. The medical management of patients with MR and atrial fibrillation is reviewed in Chapter 3.

In summary, asymptomatic patients with MR should be followed yearly with history, physical examination, and echocardiography. If symptoms develop or if ejection fraction declines to or approaches 60%

or left ventricular end-systolic dimension approaches 45 mm, the patient should be referred to a cardiologist for preoperative evaluation. Mitral valve repair is preferable to mitral valve replacement and can be performed in most patients with nonrheumatic MR. In patients with far-advanced disease, referral is indicated for assessment for surgery. Such patients may still improve, provided the mitral valve apparatus can be preserved at the time of operation.

SPECIAL CIRCUMSTANCES

Acute Mitral Regurgitation

Acute MR has a vastly different clinical presentation and prognosis than chronic MR. Because these patients may have an extremely high mortality and may die within hours of presentation, they should be referred immediately to a cardiologist and a cardiothoracic surgeon. In severe acute MR, patients may require specialized therapy with intravenous vasodilators or intraaortic balloon counterpulsation. A further discussion of this entity is beyond the intended scope of this chapter.

Mitral Valve Prolapse

Mitral valve prolapse refers to a group of conditions in which the mid-portion of one or both mitral valve leaflets "buckle" backwards behind the plane of the mitral annulus (i.e., prolapse into the left atrium) during systole. The most common pathologic cause of mitral valve relapse is myxomatous degeneration of the mitral valve. Other causes of pathologic prolapse include the Marfan syndrome and collagen vascular disease. The term mitral valve prolapse "syndrome" refers to a degenerative condition of the mitral valve in which thickened and redundant leaflets are associated with atypical chest pain at rest, autonomic dysfunction, and a modest risk of adverse events, including progression to severe MR, stroke, and infective endocarditis. Most patients with mitral valve prolapse are asymptomatic. A minority complain of atypical chest pain, palpitations, fatigue, and orthostatic lightheadedness. Asymptomatic patients generally require no therapy. Those patients who clearly have thickened and redundant mitral valve leaflets, particularly if accompanied by a murmur of MR, should undergo endocarditis prophylaxis for those procedures that cause a bacteremia, as discussed in Chapter 11.

In patients who complain of chest pain or palpitations, beta blockers, diltiazem, or verapamil may be effective therapy. A minority of patients with mitral valve prolapse are at risk for stroke. These appear to be those patients who have anatomically misshapen valves and the murmur of MR.

In patients with thickened and redundant mitral valves, daily low-dose aspirin therapy probably is indicated, although no trials have been performed to substantiate this recommendation. Finally, when mitral valve prolapse has led to severe MR, the regurgitation is treated in the same manner as described previously for the treatment of MR from any cause.

AORTIC REGURGITATION

The aortic valve may become incompetent due to pathology of either the aortic valve leaflets or the aortic root. As shown in Table 4.3, a number of diseases can cause AR, including rheumatic fever, infective endocarditis, syphilis, bicuspid aortic valve, anorectic drugs, hypertension, connective tissue diseases, aortic root dilatation (or aneurysm), aortic dissection, and trauma. Aortic regurgitation imposes a volume and a pressure overload on the heart, which in turn stimulates ventricular hypertrophy. However, unlike MR, the excess stroke volume is ejected into a high-pressure chamber, the aorta, where it increases pulse pressure. Thus, systolic hypertension frequently accompanies AR, making it a combined pressure and volume overload. As with MR, systolic function initially is preserved, but with time left ventricular systolic function declines and ultimately results in irreversible depression of the left ventricular function. Thus, as with MR, AR should be corrected before left ventricular function becomes severe and irreversible.

DIAGNOSIS OF AORTIC REGURGITATION

Symptoms

Patients with severe AR and normal left ventricular function may be remarkably asymptomatic, even during strenuous exertion. When symptoms do develop, they usually are related to left-sided congestive heart failure.

TABLE 4.3. *Causes of aortic regurgitation*

Infective endocarditis
Aortic dissection
Trauma
Hypertension
Rheumatic fever
Congenital
Syphilis
Marfan syndrome
Ankylosing spondylitis, Reiter's disease, systemic lupus erythematosus
Anorectic drugs

❂ CLINICAL PEARLS ❂

Patients with AR occasionally will develop angina pectoris in the absence of coronary disease. Angina probably develops in part due to the relative diastolic hypotension that develops due to the valve incompetence. Because the coronary arteries fill in diastole, a lowered diastolic blood pressure reduces the driving force filling the coronary arteries and reduces coronary blood flow.

Less common complaints in patients with AR include syncope, an unpleasant awareness of the heartbeat (due to the increased stroke volume), or carotid artery pulsations.

Physical Examination

In chronic AR, the apical impulse usually is displaced downward, consistent with left ventricular enlargement. The aortic component of the second heart sound often is diminished (except in hypertension and syphilis). The classic murmur of AR is best heard with the patient sitting and leaning forward with the breath held in end expiration. The murmur is typically early diastolic and decrescendo in nature, and it is heard maximally at the left sternal border in rheumatic heart disease and along the right sternal border with aortic root dilatation. As the regurgitant jet impinges on the mitral valve, it may cause partial valve closure and a low-pitched rumble of physiologic mitral stenosis (Austin Flint murmur). Peripheral signs of chronic AR (Table 4.3) reflect the increased stroke volume and include:

- Corrigan's sign: Forceful carotid pulsations
- de Musset's sign: Head bobbing with heart beat
- Quincke's pulse: Capillary pulsations, when nail bed is compressed
- Pistol shot sign: Systolic arterial sounds heard over large arteries
- Duroziez's murmur: To-and-fro murmur heard on compression (distal to site of auscultation) of large arteries
- Hill's sign: Increased blood pressure in the legs above that in the arm.

However, these signs are not specific for AR and may be detected in other diseases with a hyperdynamic state (e.g., fever, pregnancy, peripheral arteriovenous fistula, hyperthyroidism, and beriberi).

Electrocardiographic Findings

There are no diagnostic findings on the ECG that are specific for AR. However, the ECG may reveal evidence of left ventricular hypertrophy and/or conduction disturbances.

Chest X-ray Findings

The chest x-ray film will reveal a dilated LV and proximal aortic root dilation. In more advanced cases of AR, there may be left atrial, right ventricular, and right atrial enlargement (cor bovinum), with or without pulmonary congestion.

Noninvasive Studies

Two-dimensional and Doppler echocardiography are the most valuable and cost-effective tests for the initial and serial evaluation of patients with AR. Echocardiography will provide information on left ventricular size, mass, and systolic function. In addition, it may be possible to determine the etiology of the AR and the aortic root size, which have implications for surgery. Continuous-wave and color flow Doppler echocardiography provide evidence for the severity of the AR. When the technical quality of the echocardiogram precludes this assessment of left ventricular function, radionuclide ventriculography may be obtained. Exercise testing may be of value in selected cases, when doubt exists about the presence and/or severity of symptoms.

Invasive Studies

When surgery is contemplated, cardiac catheterization is indicated to (i) determine the presence or absence of coronary artery disease and (ii) confirm the echocardiographic estimate of the severity of regurgitation by aortography.

MANAGEMENT OF CHRONIC AORTIC REGURGITATION

Surgical Therapy

Correction of aortic insufficiency must be performed before the development of irreversible left ventricular dysfunction if the symptoms of heart failure are to be relieved and if the patient is to have a normal postoperative lifespan. In most cases of AR, valve replacement instead of repair is necessary (Table 4.4). Thus, in deciding when to operate, the primary care provider must weigh the risks of a prosthesis against the risk of delaying surgery. For most patients a good outcome can be expected, provided the echocardiographic left ventricular end-systolic dimension does not exceed 55 mm and that the left ventricular ejection fraction is not lower than 55%.

TABLE 4.4. *Guidelines for referral for valve replacement in aortic regurgitation*

Symptoms	ESD (mm)	EF	Course of action
None	<55	>0.55	Begin vasodilators, observe
>Mild	<55	>0.55	Refer for further evaluation
None	≥55 or	<0.55	Refer for further evaluation
Yes	≥55 or	<0.55	Refer for further evaluation

EF, ejection fraction; ESD, left ventricular end-systolic dimension.
(Adapted from Carabello BA. Recognition and management of patients with valvular heart disease. In Goldman L, Braunwald E, eds. *Primary cardiology,* 1st ed. Philadelphia: WB Saunders, 1998:383.)

❍ CLINICAL PEARLS ❍

An easy way to remember when to refer a patient for valve replacement in AR is to apply the "55" rule; that is, consider valve replacement when the echocardiographically determined left ventricular end-systolic dimension exceeds 55 mm and/or the left ventricular ejection fraction is lower than 55%.

Thus, for asymptomatic patients, operation can be delayed until either symptoms develop or the aforementioned thresholds are approached. If end-systolic diameter is less than 40 mm, it is unlikely that ventricular dysfunction will develop within 2 years, and, thus, echocardiography can be performed safely at 2-year intervals. For end-systolic diameters between 40 and 50 mm, yearly echocardiographic follow-up is recommended; if end-systolic diameter is greater than 50 mm but less than 55 mm, echocardiographic follow-up should be performed every 6 months. When symptoms of heart failure develop in a patient with severe AR, surgery should be performed regardless of the echocardiographic findings because the new onset of heart failure indicates cardiac decompensation.

After surgery, repeat echocardiography is needed for the evaluation of left ventricular size and mass, which usually regress after successful surgery, as well as for the assessment of the prosthetic valve function. The echocardiographic study should be obtained before the patient is discharged and serves as a baseline study for future comparisons. If left ventricular systolic dysfunction is present, angiotensin-converting enzyme (ACE) inhibitors may be used to forestall the development of symptomatic heart failure (see Chapter 1).

Medical Therapy

Unlike the situation with MR, vasodilator therapy in asymptomatic patients with normal left ventricular function can delay both the onset of left ventricular dysfunction as well as the need for surgery. The vasodilators that have been used thus far include nifedepine, hydralazine, and ACE inhibitors. By decreasing the peripheral vascular resistance, these drugs increase the systemic output and decrease the regurgitant volume. However, the best documentation for this effect exists for nifedipine. The current recommendations are that patients with asymptomatic AR should receive a total daily dose of 30 to 60 mg of nifedipine. If nifedipine is tolerated poorly, it is reasonable to consider the use of ACE inhibitors, hydralazine, or amlodipine. However, when symptoms develop, the ejection fraction approaches 0.55, or end-systolic diameter approaches 55 mm, patients should be referred for preoperative evaluation, as discussed earlier. For patients who are deemed as inoperable or who refuse surgery, the use of vasodilators is appropriate as a long-term strategy.

SPECIAL CIRCUMSTANCES

Acute Aortic Regurgitation

Acute AR has a vastly different clinical presentation and prognosis than chronic AR. The peripheral signs of chronic AR usually are not present because of the reduced forward stroke volume. Unequal pulses in the upper and/or lower extremities may be detected with an aortic dissection. The murmur of AR is often very brief and may not be heard at all. In patients who present with acute AR, a search should be made for possible causes of acute AR, particularly infective endocarditis or aortic dissection. When acute AR is suspected, an emergency transthoracic echocardiogram will confirm the presence and severity of AR, its etiology, and the ventricular size (usually normal) and function. When dissection is suspected, a transthoracic echocardiogram should be performed to evaluate the ascending aorta for the presence of a dissection. Therapy with nitroprusside may be attempted, because vasodilators can reduce the aortic root pressure and thus the AR volume. Immediate cardiology and cardiothoracic consultations should be obtained, as the only definitive treatment for this condition is surgery.

AORTIC STENOSIS

Aortic stenosis is the most common of the primary valvular heart diseases. Approximately 1% of Americans are born with a bicuspid aortic valve, which is the most common congenital abnormality of the heart. Of this group, a substantial proportion eventually will develop significant aortic valvular obstruction. Other patients develop stenosis of a previously normal tricuspid aortic valve. In either situation, AS is due to idiopathic degeneration and calcification of the valve. In industrialized societies, rheumatic heart disease is now a rare cause of AS.

○ CLINICAL PEARLS ○

In rheumatic AS, the mitral valve almost always is abnormal. Thus, the diagnosis of rheumatic AS should not be made in the face of an echocardiographically normal mitral valve.

Aortic stenosis results in a significant increase in afterload for the LV. The increased afterload in turn stimulates concentric left ventricular hypertrophy. At first, the left ventricular ejection fraction is normal; however, later on the ejection fraction will become depressed. This initial change in left ventricular ejection is due to the excessive afterload imposed by the stenotic aortic valve ("afterload mismatch") and is completely reversible initially. However, the hypertrophied heart eventually develops contractile dysfunction, resulting in the development of symptoms, with increased morbidity and mortality.

DIAGNOSIS OF AORTIC STENOSIS

Symptoms

A detailed history is crucial in patients with AS, because the development of symptoms in AS patients is the major indication for valve replacement. Initially, most patients with AS are asymptomatic. Survival is nearly normal during this asymptomatic phase. However, when the classic symptoms of angina, syncope, or congestive heart failure develop, there is a rapid increase in the risk of death unless aortic valve replacement is performed. Survival following the onset of angina is approximately 5 years, whereas survival following the onset of syncope or heart failure is 3 and 2 years, respectively. Sudden death usually occurs in symptomatic patients and is rarely, if ever, the first presentation of a patient with AS.

Physical Examination

The murmur of AS is typically a harsh mid-to-late peaking systolic ejection murmur that radiates to the neck. The murmur usually is heard best at the second right intercostal space, but it may be loudest close to the apex or lower left sternal border in older patients. The intensity of the aortic component of the second heart sound is diminished. In some patients, a thrill may be present at the base of the heart.

✪ CLINICAL PEARLS ✪

In hemodynamically significant AS with preserved left ventricular function, there is usually a thrill present at the base of the heart. However, in patients with severe AS and a depressed ejection fraction, the thrill may no longer be present; moreover, the murmur of AS may be only faintly audible. Thus, the absence of a thrill and a typical murmur does not exclude the presence of significant AS.

Other findings on auscultation include an ejection click (in valvular stenosis with bicuspid valves) with some valvular mobility being still present, a fourth heart sound due to impaired left ventricular relaxation, and possibly a third heart sound in patients with heart failure.

Electrocardiographic Findings

The ECG usually will reveal left ventricular hypertrophy and left atrial enlargement. There may be evidence of conduction disorders in older patients with concomitant degenerative and/or calcific disease of the conduction system.

Chest X-ray Findings

The chest x-ray film often will show a boot-shaped heart consistent with the development of left ventricular hypertrophy. Occasionally, aortic valve calcification is seen in the lateral view.

Noninvasive Studies

Two-dimensional and Doppler echocardiography provide important data about patients with AS, including aortic valve anatomy, left ventricular size and function, left ventricular hypertrophy, and pulmonary artery pressures, as well as important hemodynamic information about the severity of the aortic valve stenosis. Importantly, a complete Doppler examination can calculate transvalvular gradients, cardiac output, and aortic valve area. In general, in resting subjects who are not in heart failure, resting "peak" gradients greater than 50 mm Hg generally are associated with severe AS. Doppler echocardiography also can be used to calculate the aortic valve area. Severe AS usually is present with an area of less than 0.7cm^2, whereas moderately stenotic valves have an area 0.7 to 1 cm^2, and mildly stenotic valves are considered to be larger than 1 cm^2. In general, most patients with severe AS will be symptomatic and require aortic valve replacement.

Invasive Studies

Because most patients with AS are in an age range where concomitant coronary artery disease is likely, adult patients with AS should undergo cardiac catheterization before surgery. During this procedure, coronary angiography displays the coronary anatomy and the transvalvular gradient is confirmed by direct pressure measurement.

MANAGEMENT OF AORTIC STENOSIS

Overall Management Strategy

Table 4.5 provides an overview of the management and referral strategy for patients who present with AS. When AS is detected on physical examination in an asymptomatic patient, an echocardiogram should be performed to quantify the severity of AS. If the aortic valve area is greater than 1.0 cm^2, the patient can be followed yearly with a history and physical examination. If the aortic valve area is between 0.75 and 1.0 cm^2 in an asymptomatic patient, follow-up should be performed every 6 months. However, if the aortic valve area is between 0.75 and 1.0 cm^2 and there are equivocal symptoms of AS, then it may be prudent to refer the patient to a cardiologist for further evaluation, particularly because the echocardiographic estimate of aortic valve area may not always be precise. However, any patient who clearly develops new onset of syncope, angina, or heart failure and has an aortic valve area that is less than 1.0 cm^2 should be referred to a cardiologist for an evaluation to determine the appropriateness of aortic valve replacement. On occasion, the patient may complain of vague symptoms not typical of the classic triad of symptoms. In such cases, stress testing may be useful in assessing symptomatic status. However, exercise testing in patients with AS is controversial, must be performed with extreme caution, and therefore should be deferred to a cardiologist.

TABLE 4.5. *Guidelines for medical therapy and referral for aortic stenosis*

Symptoms	Aortic valve area (cm^2)	Course of action
None	>1.0	Observe
None	0.75–1.0	Observe every 6 months
Equivocal	<1.0	Refer for further evaluation
Angina or syncope	<1.0	Refer for further evaluation
Heart failure	Any stenosis	Refer for further evaluation
Angina or syncope	>1.0	Consider another cause
Symptomatic but aortic valve surgery contraindicated	<0.75	Consider balloon aortic valvotomy

Medical Management

There is no effective medical management for AS, aside from the use of antibiotics as prophylaxis against infective endocarditis (see Chapter 11). However, in some patients, nitrates and diuretics may be used cautiously to treat angina and heart failure, respectively, until surgery can be performed. Because patients with AS are very dependent on the left atrial contribution to left ventricular filling, it is important to maintain sinus rhythm in these patients. There are certain classes of drugs that should be avoided in patients with significant AS. Beta blockers may precipitate cardiovascular collapse and generally should be avoided in the treatment of angina. *ACE inhibitors and other vasodilators that are used for the treatment of most forms of heart failure may precipitate syncope and/or death in patients with AS.* Therefore, these agents are contraindicated.

SPECIAL CIRCUMSTANCES

Asymptomatic Aortic Stenosis

As noted earlier, asymptomatic patients with AS and preserved left ventricular function do not require aortic valve replacement. However, the primary care provider should be aware that these patients may rapidly progress to symptomatic AS. Therefore, patients with asymptomatic AS should be followed closely with a repeat history and physical examination every 6 months, with close attention paid to symptoms and signs of pulmonary congestion and/or left ventricular systolic dysfunction. In the rare circumstance where there has been a clear decrement in left ventricular function in the asymptomatic patient, aortic valve replacement is advisable. Patients who develop symptoms referable to AS should be referred to a cardiothoracic surgeon for aortic valve replacement.

Percutaneous Valvotomy

In severely symptomatic patients who are not candidates for aortic valve replacement (because of other life-limiting illnesses such as terminal cancer or severe comorbid conditions that make them nonsurgical candidates), balloon aortic valvotomy provides temporary improvement in the transvalvular gradient and may relieve symptoms in some patients. During this procedure, a large balloon catheter is advanced percutaneously from the femoral artery and over a guidewire to the aortic valve orifice. There, balloon inflation modestly increases valve cusp mobility. Unfortunately, the stenosis returns to its original severity within 6 months in approximately half of the patients in whom this procedure is attempted. Balloon aortic valvuloplasty in adults with critical, calcific AS does not lessen the high mortality rate in these patients, although it may serve as a "bridge" to valve replacement. Percutaneous valvotomy also may be considered in patients with cardiogenic shock or severe heart failure to stabilize them before undergoing definitive aortic valve replacement.

VALVE PROSTHESIS

The primary care provider should be familiar with the three types of valve prosthesis currently utilized (Table 4.6).

Bioprosthetic Heterografts

Bioprosthetic heterografts typically are made from porcine aortic valves. The advantage of these valves is that they are associated with a low risk of thromboembolism. Therefore, chronic anticoagulation with warfarin is not required. The major drawback of porcine valves is that many of these valves will have degenerated by 10 years; thus, these valves generally are not utilized in younger patients.

Mechanical Valves

The advantage of mechanical valves is their durability. Many valves can last 20 years or longer. The disadvantage of these valves is that they are thrombogenic and require chronic anticoagulation with warfarin (discussed in detail in Chapter 10). The current most commonly utilized mechanical valve is the St. Jude valve, which uses two semicircular discs. The older Starr-Edwards valve uses what is called a "ball-and cage" design.

TABLE 4.6. *Characteristics of commonly used prosthetic valves*

Valve name	Type	Anticoagulant	Durability
Carpentier-Edwards	B	No, unless large LA and AF	5–15 yr
Hancock	B	Same	5–15 yr
St. Jude	M	Yes	Unlimited
Medtronic-Hall	M	Yes	Unlimited
Starr-Edwards	M	Yes	Unlimited

AF, atrial fibrillation; B, bioprosthesis; LA, left atrium; M, mechanical valve.
(Adapted from Carabello BA. Recognition and management of patients with valvular heart disease. In Goldman L, Braunwald E, eds. *Primary cardiology,* 1st ed. Philadelphia: WB Saunders, 1998:389.)

Human Homograft Valves

Human homograft valves are sewn into the aortic position and, occasionally, can be modified for use in the mitral position. They do not require anticoagulation and seem especially resistant to endocarditis. They appear durable, although long-term follow-up is limited.

SUMMARY

Figure 4.1 provides an overview of a suggested approach to the evaluation and management of patients with valvular heart disease. The evaluation begins with a detailed history and physical examination. If the initial evaluation suggests valvular heart disease, the next step in the evaluation is to order an echocardiogram. If the noninvasive evaluation suggests significant valvular heart disease, then depending on the presence or absence of symptoms and the presence or absence of critical values on the echocardiographic evaluation, it may be appropriate to refer the patient to a cardiologist for further evaluation for valve repair and/or replacement.

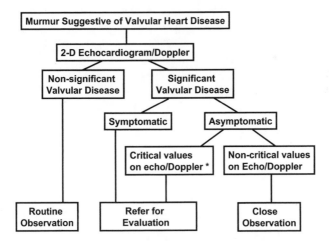

FIG. 4.1. Approach to the diagnosis and evaluation of patients with valvular heart disease. *Critical values for mitral regurgitation are given in Table 4.2; critical values for aortic regurgitation are given in Table 4.4; and critical values for aortic stenosis are given in Table 4.5.

5

Care of the Patient with Chronic Stable Angina

Glenn N. Levine

Baylor College of Medicine, Cardiac Catheterization Laboratory, Houston V. A. Medical Center, Houston, Texas 77030

Given the prevalence of coronary artery disease, most primary care providers will be involved in the care of many patients with chronic stable angina. The primary goals in these patients are to ameliorate anginal symptoms and to ensure that interventions designed to minimize the degree of coronary artery disease progression and decrease the chances of future myocardial infarction are implemented. In many cases, management of patients with chronic stable angina also includes ordering a stress test for the purposes of risk stratification. The most important management decision in patients with chronic angina involves deciding which patients should be referred for cardiac catheterization and coronary revascularization. These issues will be discussed in this chapter. An overview of the management of the patient with chronic stable angina is given in Figure 5.1.

CHRONIC STABLE ANGINA: DEFINITIONS AND CHARACTERISTICS

Angina

Angina is a *clinical diagnosis* based primarily on the patient's description of his or her symptoms. The term angina refers to the pain or discomfort a patient experiences when myocardial ischemia occurs.

✪ CLINICAL PEARLS ✪

Other causes of chronic chest-area pains that may be misinterpreted as the discomfort of chronic stable angina due to epicardial coronary artery disease include aortic stenosis, hypertrophic cardiomyopathy, syndrome X (microvascular disease), esophageal reflux, peptic ulcer disease, biliary disease, and musculoskeletal conditions.

57

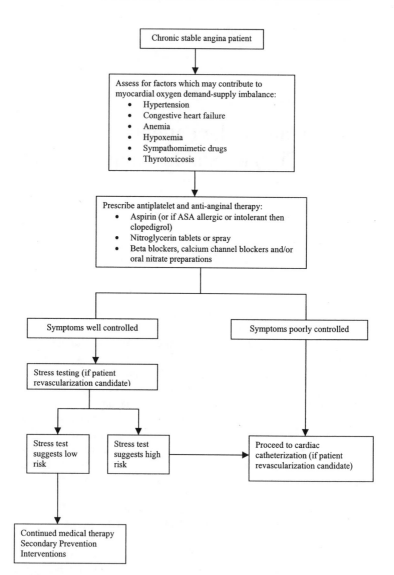

FIG. 5.1. Algorithm for the evaluation and management of patients with chronic stable angina.

Chronic Stable Angina

Chronic stable angina refers to angina that has existed on the order of months or years and which occurs at least somewhat reproducibly with comparable levels of activity (such as climbing several flights of stairs) and or with identifiable precipitants (such as with anger or after eating a large meal).

Anginal Episodes

Anginal episodes occur when myocardial oxygen demand exceeds supply. Anginal episodes usually last on the order of several to 30 minutes. Pains that last only seconds or for days are not likely to be due to angina but to a noncardiac cause. Although the majority of patients with chronic stable angina have angina associated with exertion, some patients experience angina primarily at night (nocturnal angina) or after eating large meals (postprandial angina).

ASSESSING FOR FACTORS WHICH MAY CONTRIBUTE TO MYOCARDIAL OXYGEN DEMAND-SUPPLY IMBALANCE

Although in most patients with chronic stable angina the primary problem is flow-restricting obstruction of one or more of the coronary arteries, occasionally there may be contributing causes of the patient's angina. These secondary causes warrant at least brief consideration when evaluating a patient with angina.

Hypertension

Higher blood pressures increase myocardial oxygen demand. All hypertensive patients with angina should undergo aggressive treatment to lower blood pressure to the normal range.

Congestive Heart Failure

Myocardial oxygen demand is increased in patients with symptomatic heart failure through multiple mechanisms. Aggressive treatment of heart failure with afterload reduction, diuretics, and possibly digoxin may decrease anginal episodes.

Anemia

Severe anemia decreases myocardial oxygen supply and leads to reflex cardiac tachycardia, increasing oxygen demand. It is prudent to check at least one hematocrit level during the initial evaluation of the patient with angina.

Hypoxemia

As with anemia, hypoxemia leads to decreased oxygen supply and to reflex tachycardia and increased oxygen demand. In patients with known severe lung disease or markedly abnormal pulmonary examinations, it may be prudent to check a room air oxygen saturation.

Sympathomimetic Drugs

Sympathomimetics will increase heart rate and ventricular contractility state and, thus, myocardial oxygen demand. Medications used in patients with reactive airway disease (inhaled beta agonists, theophylline) are common culprits. If possible, the use of sympathomimetics in patients with frequent anginal attacks should be minimized.

Thyrotoxicosis

Although an extremely rare contributing cause of angina, thyrotoxicosis should be considered in patients with persistent, unexplained resting tachycardia.

ACUTE ANTIANGINAL THERAPY: NITROGLYCERIN TABLETS AND SPRAYS

All patients with chronic stable angina should be prescribed nitroglycerin sublingual tablets or nitroglycerin spray. Patients should be instructed to carry the nitroglycerin with them at all times and, when an anginal attack occurs, they can take one tablet or spray every 5 minutes up to a total of three tablets or sprays. They should be instructed that if the anginal discomfort persists after three treatments, it may indicate that they are having a myocardial infarction and that they should be transported immediately to an emergency room for evaluation.

Nitroglycerin tablets come in three different doses. Most commonly, the dose of 0.4 mg (1:150 grain) is prescribed. Patients should be instructed to place the tablet under the tongue (not to swallow it!). Nitroglycerin spray is available in an aerosol preparation that delivers 0.4 mg each spray. Patients should be instructed to spray the nitroglycerin onto or under the tongue (and not to inhale the spray!).

The most important side effect of nitroglycerin therapy is hypotension. Patients should be instructed not to continue taking further doses of the nitroglycerin if they become lightheaded or dizzy. Because nitroglycerin tablets may lose their potency over time, patients should be instructed to obtain a new bottle of tablets every 6 months.

Nitroglycerin tablets or spray also may be used prophylactically before patients engage in physical activity that is likely to lead to an anginal attack. The patient should take one tablet or dose of spray 5 to 10 minutes before engaging in the activity.

CHRONIC ANTIANGINAL THERAPY

The goals of chronic antianginal therapy include increasing the amount of exertion a patient can engage without having angina, decreasing the overall frequency of anginal attacks, and minimizing the side effects of therapy.

In patients with mild exertional angina, a single antianginal agent may be adequate initial therapy. Because beta blockers have been shown to prolong life in patients after myocardial infarction, these agents seem a reasonable first choice in patients with stable coronary artery disease, particularly in those whose angina is precipitated by exertion or other activities that increase heart rate and blood pressure. In patients with normal ejection fractions and severe reactive airway disease who are unable to take beta blockers, a calcium channel blocker that slows heart rate (diltiazem or verapamil) is a reasonable alternative therapy.

In patients with continued angina on monotherapy or in patients with more severe angina and/or extensive coronary artery disease, combination therapy, such as a beta blocker and either a primarily vasodilating calcium channel blocker (such as amlodipine) or an oral nitrate preparation, should be considered.

Beta Blockers

Beta blockers decrease resting heart rate, decrease left ventricular contractility, and blunt the heart rate and blood pressure response to exercise and other physiologic stresses. In patients without contraindications to use, beta blockers should be considered first-line therapy (either as monotherapy or in combination with a second antianginal agent). Patients with overt physical findings of congestive heart failure (such as pulmonary rales) at the time of evaluation that is believed due to depressed left ventricular function should not be treated with beta blockers. Other contraindications to beta blocker use include baseline bradycardia, severe atrioventricular node conduction abnormalities, and *severe* reactive airway disease. The dose of the beta blocker should be titrated upward to achieve a resting heart rate of 50 to 60 beats/min. Side effects to inform patients about include worsening heart failure, fatigue, and impotence.

Multiple different beta blockers are available. The most commonly used beta blockers are metoprolol (Lopressor) and atenolol (Tenormin). Beta blockers that have a relative selectivity for the beta-1 receptor are, in theory, less apt to worsen pulmonary status in patients with reactive airway disease. Agents with intrinsic sympathomimetic activity may lower resting heart rate less than beta blockers without intrinsic sympathomimetic activity and thus have a role in patients with relatively slow heart rates at rest who require beta-blocker therapy. Suggested dosing regimens for selected currently available beta blockers are given in Table 5.1.

Calcium Channel Blockers

Calcium channel blockers act to varying degrees to dilate peripheral and coronary arteries, slow heart rate, and decrease left ventricular contractility. In simplified terms, verapamil and diltiazem act to a large extent to slow heart rate and decrease contractility, although they also have some vasodilating actions. Amlodipine and nifedipine act mainly as vasodilators. In general, verapamil or diltiazem should be used if beta-blocker therapy is contraindicated due to the presence of severe reactive airway disease. The primarily vasodilating calcium channel blockers can be used as a second antianginal agent in those being treated with beta blockers.

Patients with depressed ejection fractions and/or those who are in congestive heart failure should not be treated with verapamil or diltiazem. Short-acting primarily vasodilating calcium channel blockers (such as nifedipine) should not be used in the absence of a beta blocker, because these agents may cause reflex tachycardia and have been asso-

Table 5.1 *Selected beta blockers and suggested oral dosing regimens used in the treatment of chronic stable angina*

Generic name	Brand name	Initial dose	Maximum dose	Comments
Atenolol	Tenormin	50 mg q.d.	100–200 mg q.d.	Beta-1 selective
Bisoprolol	Zebeta	5 mg q.d.	20 mg q.d.	Beta-1 selective
Metoprolol	Lopressor, Toprol XL	50 mg b.i.d. 100 mg q.d.	100 mg b.i.d. 200 mg q.d.	Beta-1 selective
Pindolol	Visken	5 mg b.i.d.	20–30 mg b.i.d.	Intrinsic sympathomimetic activity
Propranolol	Inderal, Inderal LA	20 mg t.i.d.–q.i.d. 80 mg q.d.	80 mg t.i.d.–q.i.d. 320 mg q.d.	

Table 5.2. *Currently available calcium channel blockers and suggested oral dosing regimens used in the treatment of chronic stable angina*

Generic name	Brand name	Initial dose	Maximum dose	Comments
Amlodipine	Norvasc	5 mg q.d.[a]	10 mg q.d	Primarily vasodilates
Diltiazem	Cardizem	30 mg t.i.d.–q.i.d.	90 mg t.i.d.–q.i.d.	Decreases heart rate
	Cardizem SR	60 mg b.i.d.	180 mg b.i.d.	and myocardial
	Cardizem CD	180 mg q.d.	360 mg q.d.[b]	contractility also
	Dilacor XR	120 mg q.d.	360 mg q.d.	vasodilates
	Tiazac	120 mg q.d.	360 mg q.d.	
Nifedipine	Procardia XL	30 mg t.i.d.	90 mg t.i.d.	Primarily vasodilates
	Adalat CC	30 mg t.i.d.	90 mg t.i.d.	
Verapamil	Calan, Isoptin	40 mg t.i.d.	160 mg t.i.d.	Decreases heart rate
	Calan SR	120 mg b.i.d.	240 mg b.i.d.	and myocardial
	Isoptin SR	120 mg q.d.	240 mg b.i.d.	contractility; also
	Veralin	120 mg q.d.	480 mg q.d.	vasodilates

[a] Consider starting dose of 2.5 mg in frail and/or elderly patients.
[b] Maximum pill size 300 mg (therefore need to prescribe two 180-mg tablets).

ciated in several studies with increased mortality when utilized as single-agent therapy.

The dose of medication should be titrated upward based on the goal of relieving or minimizing the patient's angina and, if the patient is hypertensive, the goal of normalizing the blood pressure. Side effects to inform patients about include hypotension, peripheral edema, and worsening of heart failure. Verapamil may cause constipation, particularly in older patients. Selected currently available calcium channel blockers and dosing regimens used in the treatment of chronic stable angina are given in Table 5.2.

Nitrates

Oral nitrates act to venodilate (which decreases ventricular wall stress and thus myocardial oxygen demand) and to dilate the coronary arteries. Most commonly, these agents are used in combination with either a beta blocker or a heart-rate slowing calcium channel blocker (verapamil or diltiazem). The dose of nitrate therapy should be titrated upward based on the goal of relieving or minimizing the patient's angina. The most common side effect of these medications is headache, which sometimes can be intolerable to patients. Oral nitrates may lower blood pressure and cause hypotension. Short-, intermediate-, and long-acting preparations are available, and are listed in Table 5.3.

Table 5.3. *Oral nitrate preparations and suggested dosing regimens used in the treatment of chronic stable angina*

Generic name	Brand name	Initial dose	Maximum dose	Comments
Isosorbide dinitrate	Isordil	10 mg b.i.d.	30 mg b.i.d.	Patient should take doses in a.m. and afternoon
Isosorbide mononitrate	Ismo Monoket	20 mg b.i.d. 20 mg b.i.d.	20 mg b.i.d. 20 mg b.i.d.	Patient should take first dose in a.m. and second dose 7 h later
Isosorbide mononitrate	Imdur	30 mg q.d.	120 mg q.d.	Patient should take dose in a.m.

<0+ **CLINICAL PEARLS** +0>

The most important factor in using oral nitrate therapy is to allow a nitrate-free interval of 8 to 14 hours. Most commonly, this is accomplished by having the patient take doses of the medication only in the morning and early afternoon.

MANAGEMENT DECISIONS REGARDING STRESS TESTING

Who Should be Referred for Stress Testing

Stress testing aids in risk stratifying patients as to whether they are at low or high risk for future cardiovascular events and/or death. During the initial evaluation of a patient with chronic stable angina, ordering a stress test for the purposes of risk stratification should be considered. Patients who are found to be at low risk based on the stress test can be managed medically, provided their symptoms are adequately controlled with medications. Those patients found to be at high risk based on the stress test generally should be referred for cardiac catheterization and revascularization. It should be noted that patients who are not candidates for revascularization (such as those with severe comorbid disease or a short life expectancy, as well as those who are unwilling to consider undergoing revascularization) should not be referred for stress testing, because even if they have a result suggesting high risk, catheterization and revascularization would not be performed.

It is not necessary to delay starting treatment with antianginal medications before obtaining a stress test for the purposes of risk stratification, as whether or not the patient is on medical therapy at the time of the stress test will not significantly alter the test results as far as risk stratification is concerned.

❖ CLINICAL PEARLS ❖

Patients with unstable anginal symptoms in which angina is occurring with minimal exertion or at rest should *not* be referred for stress testing, as it is possible that the stress test might provoke a severe episode of myocardial ischemia or even a myocardial infarction.

Choosing the Appropriate Stress Test

In most patients, exercise treadmill testing with electrocardiographic monitoring is recommended as the test of choice. In some patients, interpretation of the electrocardiogram will be unreliable, and such patients should be referred for an imaging study (either a nuclear imaging study with thallium or the newer agent "sestaMIBI," or an echocardiographic study). Conditions that interfere with interpretation of the electrocardiogram and for which patients should be referred for an imaging study are listed in Table 5.4. Patients referred for nuclear imaging or echocardiographic studies should be referred for exercise treadmill studies (as opposed to pharmacologic stress studies), unless they are unable to exercise.

❖ CLINICAL PEARLS ❖

The standard exercise treadmill study is called the Bruce protocol, in which every 3 minutes the speed and incline of the treadmill increase. Each 3-minute period is called a stage. Patients who are unable to complete the first 3 minutes of the protocol (stage 1) for whatever reason have a poorer prognosis, whereas those who complete 9 minutes of the protocol (stage 3) have a good overall prognosis.

In patients who are unable to exercise, a pharmacologic stress is utilized. When nuclear imaging is utilized, persantine is the usual agent. Persantine dilates the coronary arteries and can lead to relative perfusion defects that can be seen between areas of the left ventricle supplied by nondiseased arteries and those supplied by diseased arteries. When

Table 5.4. *Factors that make interpretation of the electrocardiogram unreliable during stress testing*

- Digoxin therapy
- Left ventricular hypertrophy
- Baseline ST depression
- Left bundle branch block
- Ventricular paced rhythm

Patients with any of these factors should be referred for imaging studies.

Table 5.5. *Criteria associated with a poorer prognosis in patients undergoing stress testing*

Exercise stress testing
- Development of angina, particularly if it occurs at a low work load (<3 min on a standard exercise test) and requires test termination
- Fall in systolic blood pressure with exercise
- ST-segment depression in ≥5 leads
- ST-segment depression ≥2 mm
- ST-segment depression lasting ≥5 min into recovery

Nuclear imaging ("thallium" or "sestaMIBI" testing)
- Multiple areas of reversible ischemia
- Increased lung uptake of thallium (indicating severe left ventricular dysfunction and/or diffuse myocardial ischemia)

echocardiography is utilized to image the heart, graded infusion of dobutamine is used to stress the heart.

Interpreting Stress Test Results

Criteria have been established for interpretation of stress tests that can distinguish patients at low risk from those at high risk. These criteria are listed in Table 5.5. Patients whose stress test results demonstrate one or more of these criteria generally should be referred for cardiac catheterization.

✪ CLINICAL PEARLS ✪

A fall in blood pressure during exercise testing is associated with the presence of severe three vessel and/or left main coronary artery disease. This finding is considered an absolute indication for cardiac catheterization.

WHEN TO REFER PATIENTS FOR CARDIAC CATHETERIZATION AND REVASCULARIZATION

Who to Refer for Cardiac Catheterization

There are, in general, two groups of patients who should be referred for cardiac catheterization and possible revascularization. The first group is those patients who, despite medical therapy, continue to have symptoms that significantly interfere with their quality of life. Such patients desire to have less frequent anginal episodes and/or to be able to engage in a greater degree of physical activity than what they are currently able to do. The second group of patients, as discussed earlier, are those with stress tests in whom the results of that stress test suggest that the patient is at high risk for future cardiovascular events.

Only patients who are candidates for revascularization should be referred for cardiac catheterization. Patients with severe comorbid disease or extremely short life expectancy, and those who are unwilling to undergo a revascularization procedure, should not be referred for catheterization, because the results of the catheterization itself, without a revascularization procedure, would not change symptoms or prognosis.

Who to Refer for Revascularization

Patients with clinical indications for revascularization (poorly controlled symptoms, markedly positive stress tests) and coronary anatomy amenable to revascularization should be referred for consideration for revascularization. Discussion with an invasive cardiologist may help to establish if the diseased vessel or vessels are amenable to percutaneous revascularization and/or bypass surgery.

Mode of Revascularization

Patients with single vessel coronary artery disease usually can be treated with percutaneous revascularization. Several large studies have demonstrated that patients with multivessel coronary artery disease may be treated with either percutaneous revascularization or bypass surgery. Management decisions in this latter group of patients may depend, in part, on technical issues and, in part, on patient preference. Issues regarding revascularization decisions are discussed in detail in Chapter 12.

SECONDARY PREVENTION

In addition to controlling the patient's angina, several important interventions that decrease the risk of coronary artery disease progression and future cardiac events should be considered in patients with chronic stable angina. These secondary prevention interventions are summarized in Table 5.6.

Aspirin and Antiplatelet Therapy

Antiplatelet therapy has been shown in multiple patient populations to decrease the incidence of future cardiovascular events and/or death. Therefore, *all patients* except those with *true* aspirin allergies should be treated with aspirin 160 to 324 mg daily (usually 324-mg enteric-coated

Table 5.6. *Secondary prevention interventions that should be considered in patients with chronic stable angina*

---

1. Antiplatelet therapy
   - Aspirin: 324 mg enteric-coated aspirin p.o. q.d.
   - Clopidogrel: 75 mg p.o. q.d.
2. Cholesterol reduction
   - In patients with LDL≥100–130 mg/dl, treat with diet and medications
   - Goal in such patients is LDL <100 mg/dl
3. Smoking cessation
   - Sternly inform patients they can no longer smoke
   - Inform patients of benefits of smoking cessation
   - Devise concrete plan and date for smoking cessation
4. Exercise
   - Discuss with patient plan for appropriate level of regular aerobic exercise

---

LDL, low-density lipoprotein.

aspirin daily). Aspirin-allergic (and probably aspirin-intolerant) patients should be treated with the potent platelet inhibitor clopidogrel (Plavix) 75 mg by mouth q.d. At the time of this writing, separate studies are currently underway to assess if the combination of aspirin plus clopidogrel is superior to aspirin alone in decreasing future ischemic events.

Cholesterol Reduction

All patients with coronary artery disease should have a complete fasting lipid profile. In patients with elevated low-density lipoprotein levels, diet and pharmacologic therapy (usually with a 3-hydroxy-3-methylglutaryl coenzyme A reductase inhibitor or "statin") should be initiated with the goal of reducing the low-density lipoprotein level to less than 100 mg/dL. Evaluation and treatment of hypercholesterolemia is discussed in detail in Chapter 9.

Estrogen Replacement Therapy

Although extensive epidemiologic data suggested beneficial effects of estrogen replacement therapy on cardiovascular disease in post-menopausal women and those who have undergone oophorectomy, a large recent study found no benefit and perhaps even an early increase in cardiovascular events in women with cardiovascular disease who were started on estrogen replacement therapy for the purposes of secondary prevention. Therefore, at the time of this writing, the current recommendation is that patients should not be started on estrogen replacement therapy for the purpose of secondary prevention. Those already on therapy can be maintained on it, and those who have other (noncardiac) indications for estrogen replacement therapy also should be treated with estrogens. A second large study of estrogens in secondary prevention is in progress at this time, and the results of this study may impact future recommendations.

Smoking Cessation

Patients with coronary artery disease cannot smoke. This statement should be told directly to the patient and spouse in no uncertain terms. The patient should be informed that within 1 year of smoking cessation the risk of myocardial infarction may decrease to half that if he or she continued smoking, and within 10 years it may decrease to approximately that of those who have not smoked. Devise with the patient a plan and date for smoking cessation.

Exercise

Regular aerobic exercise can increase the time a patient can exert themselves before developing angina (the training effect), have modest beneficial effects on cholesterol profile, blood pressure, and weight status, and may lead to an overall decrease in future cardiovascular events and mortality. These benefits and a plan for moderate aerobic exercise should be discussed with patients.

SUMMARY

Chronic stable angina is a clinical diagnosis based on the patient's description of anginal symptoms that have occurred for months or years and are predominantly reproducible with comparable levels of activity and/or identifiable precipitants. Anginal episodes occur when myocardial oxygen demand exceeds supply. Factors that may be contributing to a myocardial oxygen demand-supply imbalance, many of which can be easily treated, should be investigated during an evaluation of the patient with chronic stable angina. Antianginal therapy consists of nitroglycerin tablets or spray administered as the occasion requires and one or more antianginal agents. Beta-blocker therapy by itself or in combination with either a vasodilating calcium channel blocker or with an oral nitrate preparation is adequate therapy in many patients with chronic stable angina. Stress testing for risk stratification should be considered in patients who are candidates for revascularization. Patients who, despite medical therapy, continue to have symptoms that significantly interfere with their quality of life and patients with stress tests that suggest they are at high risk for future cardiac events should be referred for cardiac catheterization, as long as the patient is a candidate for revascularization. Secondary prevention interventions, including the use of aspirin or other antiplatelet agents, cholesterol reduction therapy, and estrogen replacement therapy, should be considered in all patients with chronic stable angina.

6

Care of the Patient with Unstable Angina

Glenn N. Levine

Baylor College of Medicine, Cardiac Catheterization Laboratory, Houston V. A. Medical Center, Houston, Texas 77030

The term *unstable angina* encompasses a spectrum of syndromes including (i) new-onset exertional angina, (ii) worsening of chronic stable angina (i.e., angina occurring more frequently or with lesser degrees of exertion), and (iii) angina that is occurring at rest. Although all of these conditions warrant concern, it is angina that is occurring at rest, without clear precipitant, that should most concern the primary care provider. In such cases, it is believed that an underlying atherosclerotic plaque has "ruptured" and become "unstable," and that intermittent thrombus formation, as well as possible coronary vasoconstriction, is occurring, decreasing myocardial oxygen supply and causing angina. The obvious concern is that at some point these episodes of transient reduction in blood flow will become fixed, leading to acute myocardial infarction. The occurrence of unstable angina that requires hospitalization is associated with at least a 10% risk of subsequent myocardial infarction if not properly treated.

DIAGNOSIS

Unstable angina is a *clinical diagnosis,* based primarily on the patient's symptoms. Although abnormalities noted on the electrocardiogram (ECG) may help corroborate the diagnosis of unstable angina, they are not necessary to such a diagnosis.

Symptoms

Typically, patients report one or more relatively brief (i.e., less than 30 minutes) anginal episodes. The practitioner should be aware that although many patients will report experiencing "classic" chest heaviness or pressure, some may instead experience only pain in the arm, neck, or jaw, or only symptoms of dyspnea, diaphoresis, or nausea. Many patients will downplay their symptoms. Therefore, the practitioner should aggressively probe the symptoms during the initial patient evaluation.

⟨⟩ CLINICAL PEARLS ⟨⟩

Some episodes of transient myocardial ischemia, particularly those associated with stenoses in the left circumflex artery, do not lead to overt abnormalities on the ECG. The lack of electrocardiographic abnormalities in a patient whose clinical history is highly suggestive of unstable angina should not be used to rule out the possibility that the patient's chest pain is caused by myocardial ischemia.

Electrocardiographic Findings

The baseline ECG in many patients who report recent symptoms suggestive of unstable angina may be normal, and such a finding does not rule out the diagnosis of unstable angina. Electrocardiographic abnormalities obtained during an episode of chest discomfort that support the diagnosis of unstable angina, particularly if these abnormalities are new compared to old or baseline ECGs, include ST-segment depression (or transient elevation) and T-wave inversions (particularly deep, symmetric T-wave inversions).

⟨⟩ CLINICAL PEARLS ⟨⟩

Other important causes of chest pain that should at least be considered in patients who present with unprovoked chest pain include aortic dissection, pneumothorax, pulmonary embolus, esophageal rupture, or peptic ulcer disease.

INITIAL OUTPATIENT MANAGEMENT CONSIDERATIONS

In patients seen in an outpatient setting who complain of chest pains and are deemed likely to have unstable angina, the first important consideration is whether the patient needs to be hospitalized. This decision is based on whether the patient is classified as having either a short-term "low risk" or "high risk" of nonfatal myocardial infarction or cardiac death.

Lower-risk Patients

Patients who are judged to be at "lower risk" may be started on medical therapy and scheduled for follow-up evaluation within 1 week. Lower-risk patients may include those with:

- Recent-onset (within the past 2 weeks to 2 months) exertional angina (without rest angina)
- Worsening of chronic exertional angina (i.e., angina that occurs more frequently or with less strenuous exertion).

Higher-risk Patients

Patients who should be considered at higher risk and consequently should be promptly hospitalized include those with:

- New-onset (within the past 2 weeks) moderate or severe angina
- Prolonged, severe episodes of angina
- Episodes of rest angina
- Dynamic ST-segment depression or T-wave inversion on an ECG that is obtained during an anginal episode
- New "ischemic-appearing" ST-segment depressions or T-wave inversions on the ECG obtained during the current evaluation.

OUTPATIENT MANAGEMENT OF LOW-RISK PATIENTS

Patients deemed at lower risk who are to have initial outpatient management should be started on aspirin, prescribed sublingual nitroglycerin tablets, and antianginal medications. First-line antianginal medications should include a beta blocker and oral nitrates. With patients already taking antianginal agents, the practitioner should increase doses of these agents or add a calcium channel blocker. The patient should undergo evaluation with stress testing for risk stratification within 3 days after medical therapy is initiated.

Aspirin

All patients except those with *true* aspirin allergies (e.g., hives, bronchospasms, anaphylaxis) should be started on aspirin, 160 to 324 mg per day (usually 324-mg enteric-coated aspirin). Aspirin-allergic patients should be started on the antiplatelet agents at a dose of 75 mg q.d. Suggested dosing regimens for aspirin and aspirin substitutes are provided in Table 6.1.

Table 6.1. *Suggested treatment regimens for outpatients with unstable angina*

Aspirin and aspirin substitutes in patients with true aspirin allergies
- Aspirin 160–324 mg p.o. q.d. (most commonly 324-mg enteric-coated acetyl-salicylic acid
- Clopidogrel (Plavix) 75 mg p.o. q.d.

Beta blockers
- Metoprolol (Lopressor) 50 mg p.o. b.i.d. initially, titrated up to a maximum of 100 mg p.o. b.i.d.. Alternately, can prescribe long-acting once-a-day Toprol XL 100 mg p.o. q.d. initially, titrated up to a maximum of 200 mg p.o. q.d.
- Atenolol (Tenormin) 50 mg p.o. q.d. initially, titrated up to a usual maximum of 100 mg p.o. q.d..

Nitrates
- Isosorbide dinitrate (Isordil) 10 mg p.o. b.i.d. or t.i.d. initially, increased up to a usual dose of 20–30 mg p.o. b.i.d. or t.i.d.
- Ismo (a longer-acting isosorbide mononitrate preparation) 20 mg p.o. b.i.d. with the patient told to take the first dose on awakening and the second dose 7 h later.
- Imdur (a long-acting isosorbide mononitrate preparation) 30 mg p.o. q.d. initially, titrated up to a maximum of 120 mg p.o. q.d..

Calcium channel blockers
- Verapamil (Calan, Isoptin) 40 mg p.o. t.i.d. initially, titrated upward as tolerated to a usual dose of 80–120 mg p.o. t.i.d.. Alternately, can prescribe long-acting once-a-day preparations (Calan SR, Isoptin SR, Veralin, Covera HS) 120 mg p.o. q.d. initially, titrated up to maximum of 360 mg p.o. q.d.. Covera HS should be prescribed to be taken in the evening.
- Diltiazem (Cardizem) 30 mg p.o. t.i.d. or q.i.d. initially, titrated upward as tolerated to a usual dose of 60–90 mg p.o. t.i.d. or q.i.d.. Alternately, can prescribe long-acting once-a-day preparations (Cardizem CD, Dilacor XR, Tiazac) 120 mg p.o. q.d. initially, titrated up to a maximum of approximately 360 mg p.o. q.d..
- Amlodipine (Norvasc) 5 mg p.o. q.d. initially (2.5 mg in frail or elderly patients), titrated upward as needed to a maximum of 10 mg p.o. q.d..

Beta Blockers

Patients without contraindications should be started on beta-blocker therapy. Patients who are in congestive heart failure at the time of presentation should not be started on beta blockers until this condition is treated. Other contraindications to beta-blocker therapy include baseline bradycardia, severe atrioventricular node conduction abnormalities, and *severe* reactive airway disease. The dose of the beta blocker should be titrated upward to achieve a resting heart rate of 50 to 60 beats/min. Side effects that patients should be told about include worsening heart failure, fatigue, and impotence. The most commonly used beta blockers are metoprolol

(Lopressor, Toprol XL) and atenolol (Tenormin). Suggested beta-blocker regimens are provided in Table 6.1.

Nitrates

Outpatients should be prescribed sublingual nitroglycerin as needed and be instructed on its use. Patients also should be started on oral nitrate therapy. Some suggested nitrate regimens are listed in Table 6.1. Patients should be advised of common side effects of nitrate therapy, particularly headache and hypotension.

Calcium Channel Blockers

Calcium channel blockers should be prescribed for patients who either cannot tolerate beta blockers or nitrates, or who continue to have angina despite maximal treatment with beta blockers and nitrates. Patients who cannot be prescribed beta blockers because of the presence of severe reactive airway disease should receive a prescription for a calcium channel blocker that slows the heart rate (diltiazem or verapamil). Patients should be advised about side effects such as constipation (with verapamil), lower-extremity edema (particularly with nifedipine and amlodipine), and hypotension. Commonly used agents and dosing regimens are listed in Table 6.1.

Stress Testing

A stress test should be scheduled for further risk stratification. In patients taking digoxin or with ECGs that demonstrate baseline ST-segment abnormalities, left ventricular hypertrophy, or left bundle branch block, interpretation of ST-segment changes is impaired. These patients need to undergo cardiac imaging as part of the stress test. Patients unable to exercise should undergo a pharmacologic stress test (such as a persantine thallium test). Criteria have been established that enable interpretation of the stress test so as to determine whether the patient is at high risk of future cardiac events or cardiac-related death. Such criteria are listed in Table 6.2.

❏ CLINICAL PEARLS ❏

Patients who experience angina with minimal exertion or at rest should not be referred for stress testing, as it is possible that the stress test itself might provoke a myocardial infarction.

Table 6.2. *Criteria associated with a poorer prognosis in patients undergoing stress testing*

Exercise stress testing
- Development of angina, particularly if it occurs at a low work load (<3 min on a standard exercise test) and requires test termination
- Fall in systolic blood pressure with exercise
- ST-segment depression in ≥5 leads
- ST-segment depression ≥2 mm
- ST-segment depression lasting ≥5 min into recovery

Nuclear imaging ("thallium" or "sestaMIBI" testing)
- Multiple areas of reversible ischemia
- Increased lung uptake of thallium (indicating severe left ventricular dysfunction and/or diffuse myocardial ischemia)

Follow-up Care

Patients whose symptoms are well controlled and who have stress test results that do not suggest that they are at high risk should be continued on medical therapy. Patients with continued or worsening symptoms and those with stress tests that suggest that they are at high risk should be referred for prompt cardiac catheterization. An algorithm for the initial evaluation and management of outpatients with symptoms of unstable angina is shown in Fig. 6.1.

INITIAL INPATIENT MANAGEMENT

Patients with higher-risk features, particularly those with episodes of rest angina and/or dynamic ST-segment changes, should receive aggressive treatment. Current standard-of-care therapy includes aspirin, heparin, and antianginal agents. Platelet glycoprotein IIb/IIIa inhibitors also should be considered in the treatment of high-risk patients. As with outpatient therapy, the preferred initial antianginal agents are beta blockers and nitrates. Calcium channel blockers should be prescribed for patients unable to tolerate beta blockers or nitrates, and for patients who have recurrent anginal episodes despite adequate beta-blocker and nitrate therapy.

Initial Patient Triage

Patients who require hospitalization but are relatively stable can be admitted to an intermediate care unit with telemetry monitoring. Patients who should be admitted for intensive treatment in a cardiac care unit include those with prolonged chest pain, ongoing chest pain, or both; dynamic ST-segment changes or "ischemic-appearing" ST or T-wave abnormalities; or ischemic pulmonary edema.

Initial Nonpharmacologic Measures

The patients should be placed on bed rest, and supplemental nasal cannula oxygen should be ordered. In patients with one or more prolonged episodes of angina, total creatine phosphokinase (CPK) and creatine phosphokinase-myoglobin (CPK-MB) levels should be obtained every 8 hours for 24 hours. Follow-up ECGs should be obtained for at least the first several days after admission and carefully assessed for new ischemic changes.

⟡ CLINICAL PEARLS ⟡

Either a troponin I or troponin T level may be obtained on admission of the patient and again approximately eight hours later. These serum assays are more sensitive than CPK measurements for determining the presence of myocardial necrosis, and elevated levels (troponin I greater than 0.4 ng/mL; troponin T greater than 0.1 ng/mL) correlate well with a greater risk of short-term adverse outcome.

Pharmacologic Measures

Aspirin

All patients except those truly allergic to aspirin should be treated with aspirin (160 to 324 mg daily). Those with true aspirin allergies can be treated with the antiplatelet agent clopidogrel (Plavix) as outlined in Table 6.3.

Beta Blockers

Patients without contraindications should be started on beta-blocker therapy. Contraindications to beta-blocker therapy include baseline bradycardia, severe atrioventricular node conduction abnormalities, active congestive heart failure, and *severe* reactive airway disease. Patients with active, ongoing ischemia should be treated initially with intravenous beta blockers such as metoprolol (Lopressor) or atenolol (Tenormin).

Nitrates

All patients except those with overt hypotension should be started on nitrate therapy. Patients with active, ongoing chest pain and those with dynamic electrocardiographic changes should be started on intravenous nitroglycerin therapy. Patients not requiring intravenous nitroglycerin most commonly are started on topical nitrates. Patients who stabilize and remain stable for several days can be switched to oral nitrate therapy. One

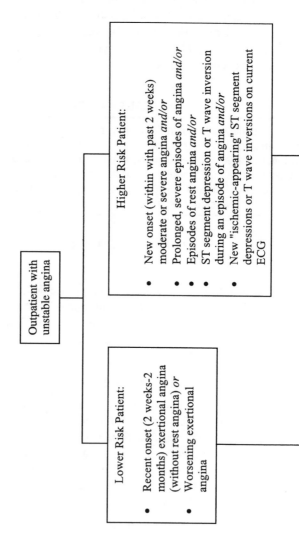

Outpatient with unstable angina

Lower Risk Patient:

- Recent onset (2 weeks-2 months) exertional angina (without rest angina) *or*
- Worsening exertional angina

Higher Risk Patient:

- New onset (within with past 2 weeks) moderate or severe angina *and/or*
- Prolonged, severe episodes of angina *and/or*
- Episodes of rest angina *and/or*
- ST segment depression or T wave inversion during an episode of angina *and/or*
- New "ischemic-appearing" ST segment depressions or T wave inversions on current ECG

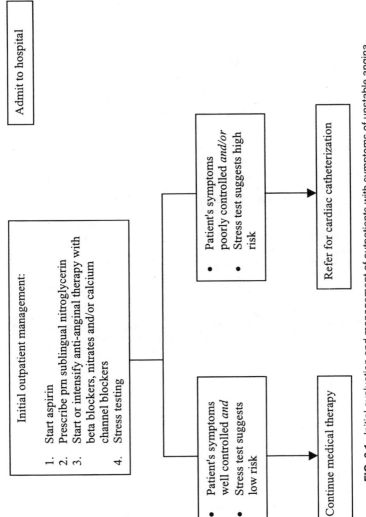

FIG. 6.1. Initial evaluation and management of outpatients with symptoms of unstable angina.

Table 6.3. *Suggested treatment regimens for inpatients with unstable angina*

Aspirin and aspirin substitutes in patients with true aspirin allergies
- Aspirin 160–324 mg p.o. q.d. (most commonly 324 mg regular aspirin initially and then 324 mg enteric-coated acetylsalicylic acid p.o. q.d.
- Clopidogrel (Plavix) 75 mg p.o. q.d. (consider a 300-mg "loading dose")

Beta blockers
- If ongoing angina and/or dynamic ST-segment changes: metoprolol (Lopressor) 5 mg IV q5min. as tolerated for a total dose of 15 mg, then either metoprolol 50 mg p.o. b.i.d. initially, titrated up to achieve a resting heart rate of 50–60 beats/min, up to a maximum dose of 100 mg p.o. b.i.d.
- Atenolol (Tenormin) 50 mg p.o. q.d. initially, titrated up to achieve a resting heart rate of 50–60 beats/min, up to a maximum dose of 100 mg p.o. q.d.

Nitrates
- If ongoing angina and/or dynamic ST-segment changes: IV nitroglycerin 10–20 μg/min initially, titrated upward as tolerated by blood pressure and as clinically indicated
- If relatively stable: nitropaste 1–2 inches q6h

Calcium channel blockers
- Verapamil (Calan, Isoptin, etc.) 40 mg p.o. t.i.d. initially, titrated upward as tolerated to a usual dose of 80–120 mg p.o. t.i.d.
- Diltiazem (Cardizem, etc.) 30 mg p.o. t.i.d. or q.i.d. initially, titrated upward as tolerated to a usual dose of 60–90 mg p.o. t.i.d. or q.i.d.
- Amlodipine:(Norvasc) 5 mg p.o. q.d. initially (2.5 mg in frail or elderly patients) titrated upward as needed to a maximum of 10 mg p.o. q.d.

Heparin
- Standard (unfractionated) heparin 80 U/kg IV bolus then 18 Ukg/h continuous IV infusion
- Low-molecular-weight heparin (such as enoxaparin [Lovenox] 1 mg/kg s.c. q12h)

Platelet IIb/IIIa receptor inhibitors
- Eptifibatide (Integrilin) 180 μg/kg bolus then 2 μg/kg/min continuous infusion for up to 72 h (Note: dose is in micrograms, not milligrams).
- Aggrastat (Tirofiban) initial infusion of 0.4 μg/kg/min IV for 30 min then continuous intravenous infusion at 0.1 μg/kg/min (Note: dose is in micrograms, not milligrams).

regimen utilizes isosorbide dinitrate (Isordil). It consists of an initial dose of 10 mg two or three times a day taken orally, titrated up to 20 to 30 mg two or three times a day taken orally. Table 6.3 lists suggested treatment regimens.

Calcium Channel Blockers

Calcium channel blockers should be prescribed for patients who either cannot tolerate beta blockers or nitrates, or who continue to have angina despite treatment with beta blockers and nitrates. Calcium channel blockers can be added to the antianginal regimens of patients who remain hypertensive. Patients who cannot be prescribed beta blockers because of the presence of severe reactive airway disease should be prescribed a calcium channel blocker that slows the heart rate (diltiazem or verapamil). Commonly used agents and their dosing regimens are listed in Table 6.3.

Heparin

The practitioner should use anticoagulation therapy with a heparin preparation *in addition* to aspirin therapy, because combining these agents is superior to using either agent alone, and bleeding complications are not significantly increased. Standard (unfractionated) heparin or low-molecular-weight heparin may be used.

The suggested regimen for standard (unfractionated) heparin is an initial intravenous bolus of 80 U/kg followed by a continuous intravenous infusion at an initial rate of 18 U/kg/h. Partial thromboplastin time (PTT) should be checked approximately 6 hours after this initial regimen, 6 hours after dose infusion changes, and then every 24 hours. Intravenous heparin infusion levels should be adjusted to maintain the PTT at 1.5 to 2.5 times control. Therapy should be continued for 2 to 5 days.

An alternative to intravenous administration of unfractionated heparin is the subcutaneous administration of low-molecular-weight heparin. Two studies have now demonstrated that one low-molecular-weight heparin, enoxaparin (Lovenox), can reduce the incidence of adverse ischemic events to a greater degree than unfractionated heparin. Additionally, low-molecular-weight heparin can be administered subcutaneously twice daily, and the PTT does not need to be monitored. Table 6.3 lists suggested treatment regimens.

Platelet IIb/IIIa Receptor Inhibitors

Recent studies demonstrated that the use of medications that block the platelet IIb/IIIa receptor and inhibit platelet aggregation provide benefits in the reduction of adverse events (death, myocardial infarction, recurrent ischemia) in patients with unstable angina above that obtained with aspirin and unfractionated heparin alone. These agents may be considered in patients who present with ST-segment depression or T-wave inversions that are believed to be due to ischemia, and in patients with positive troponin or creatine kinase-myoglobin (CK-MB) levels. If platelet IIb/IIIa inhibitors are given, they should be used in addition to standard therapy, including aspirin, unfractionated heparin, and antianginal agents. Currently approved agents include eptifibatide (Integrilin) and tirofiban (Aggrastat). Suggested dosing regimens are listed in Table 6.3.

Eptifibatide (Integrilin): Administer an 180 μg/kg bolus, then a continuous infusion of 2 μg/kg/min for up to 72 hours. Treat with aspirin and intravenous heparin (with target PTT of 50 to 75 seconds). Eptifibatide should not be used with patients with creatinine levels above 2.0 mg/dL.

Tirofiban (Aggrastat): Administer an initial 0.4 µg/kg/min intravenously for 30 minutes, then a continuous intravenous infusion at 0.1 µg/kg/min. Treat with aspirin and intravenous heparin (with target PTT approximately two times control). Patients with severely impaired renal function should receive half the usual initial loading dose and half the usual continuous infusion rate. Check platelet count within 6 hours following administrations of loading infusion and daily thereafter watching for the rare development of thrombocytopenia.

A third agent, *abciximab (ReoPro),* is currently undergoing study (GUSTO IV–ACS) in patients with acute coronary syndromes.

Contraindications to the use of IIb/IIIa inhibitors vary slightly from agent to agent, but generally include those factors that predispose patients to increased bleeding risks, including prior intracranial hemorrhage or history of recent stroke of any kind, recent or ongoing bleeding, recent major surgery or trauma, severe hypertension, or below-normal platelet count. Before using IIb/IIIa inhibitors, the practitioner should consult the manufacturer's instructions enclosed with the medication for a full listing of contraindications.

FOLLOW-UP INPATIENT CARE: DECIDING BETWEEN CARDIAC CATHETERIZATION AND CONSERVATIVE THERAPY

An important management decision with hospitalized patients who have unstable angina is determining whether they should be referred for cardiac catheterization or instead be managed with an initial conservative strategy of medical therapy and predischarge stress testing.

When to Refer Patients for Cardiac Catheterization

Several studies of patients with unstable angina have been conducted that have compared two treatment strategies: (i) initial medical therapy and predischarge testing, with catheterization and revascularization reversed for only those with recurrent or inducible angina; and (ii) early cardiac catheterization and revascularization. One study found a slight advantage over this early invasive strategy; a second study found the two strategies lead to similar outcomes. Therefore, in many patients, the choice between the two strategies can be based, at least partly, on patient preference. Patients who clearly should be referred for cardiac catheterization (with an eye toward revascularization) include those with (i) recurrent spontaneous angina despite medical therapy, (ii) a positive predischarge stress test, and (iii) ischemic pulmonary edema.

Continued Medical Therapy and Stress Testing

In instances when the practitioner elects to try an initial conservative strategy of medical therapy and predischarge stress testing, heparin therapy can be discontinued after 2 to 5 days if the patient has remained stable and has experienced no further angina. If there is no further angina for 24 hours after cessation of heparin therapy, the patient should undergo a predischarge stress test. In patients on digoxin or with ECGs that demonstrate baseline ST-segment abnormalities, left ventricular hypertrophy, or left bundle branch block, interpretation of ST-segment changes is impaired. These patients need to have cardiac imaging (such as a thallium study) as part of the stress test. Patients unable to exercise should undergo a pharmacologic stress test (most commonly a persantine thallium or dobutamine echo test). Patients with "positive" stress tests (i.e., tests that show inducible angina, marked ST-segment changes, large or multiple areas of reversible ischemia on the imaging study) should be referred for cardiac catheterization (Fig. 6.2).

POSTDISCHARGE CARE

Patients should be seen several weeks after discharge for follow-up. At that time, the practitioner should determine if symptoms have recurred or worsened. During this visit, the practitioner and patient should discuss secondary prevention measures, including smoking cessation and cholesterol reduction. The practitioner and the patient also should discuss and plan a program of aerobic exercise.

SUMMARY

Unstable angina is a *clinical diagnosis,* based primarily on the patient's symptoms. Patients with recent-onset exertional angina and those with chronic exertional angina that has worsened often can be managed initially as outpatients. Those patients with new-onset moderate or severe angina, prolonged or severe episodes of angina, episodes of rest angina, dynamic ST-segment or T-wave changes with anginal episodes, or new ST-segment or T-wave abnormalities on an ECG obtained at the time of evaluation should be promptly hospitalized. Outpatient management includes prescribing aspirin, sublingual nitroglycerin as required, and antianginal medications, and scheduling a stress test for risk stratification. Hospitalized patients should be treated with aspirin, heparin, and aggressive

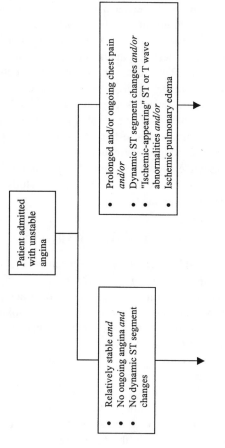

Patient admitted with unstable angina

- Relatively stable *and*
- No ongoing angina *and*
- No dynamic ST segment changes

- Prolonged and/or ongoing chest pain *and/or*
- Dynamic ST segment changes *and/or*
- "Ischemic-appearing" ST or T wave abnormalities *and/or*
- Ischemic pulmonary edema

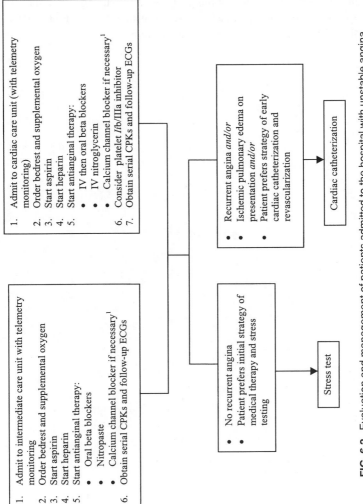

FIG. 6.2. Evaluation and management of patients admitted to the hospital with unstable angina.

Admit to intermediate care unit with telemetry monitoring box:

1. Admit to intermediate care unit with telemetry monitoring
2. Order bedrest and supplemental oxygen
3. Start aspirin
4. Start heparin
5. Start antianginal therapy:
   - Oral beta blockers
   - Nitropaste
   - Calcium channel blocker if necessary[1]
6. Obtain serial CPKs and follow-up ECGs

Admit to cardiac care unit box:

1. Admit to cardiac care unit (with telemetry monitoring)
2. Order bedrest and supplemental oxygen
3. Start aspirin
4. Start heparin
5. Start antianginal therapy:
   - IV then oral beta blockers
   - IV nitroglycerin
   - Calcium channel blocker if necessary[1]
6. Consider platelet *Ib/IIIa* inhibitor
7. Obtain serial CPKs and follow-up ECGs

- No recurrent angina
- Patient prefers initial strategy of medical therapy and stress testing

Stress test

- Recurrent angina *and/or*
- Ischemic pulmonary edema on presentation *and/or*
- Patient prefers strategy of early cardiac catheterization and revascularization

Cardiac catheterization

antianginal therapy, and they should be considered for treatment with a IIb/IIIa inhibitor. Whether inpatients should be referred for cardiac catheterization depends, in part, on patient preference and on whether the patient has recurrent angina or presents with ischemic pulmonary edema. Inpatients managed with an initial conservative strategy of medical therapy should undergo predischarge stress testing; those who test positive should be referred for cardiac catheterization.

7

Management of the Patient with Myocardial Infarction

Glenn N. Levine

Baylor College of Medicine, Cardiac Catheterization Laboratory, Houston V. A. Medical Center, Houston, Texas 77030

Acute myocardial infarction (MI) continues to be the leading cause of death in the United States. Each year, approximately 900,000 Americans suffer acute MI, and approximately one fourth of these persons die. Whereas in the past, care for patients with acute MI was mostly supportive, over the last decade there has been a great deal of research into interventions that can decrease the extent of infarcted myocardium, improve resultant left ventricular function, and decrease mortality. Recommended management of patients with MI, from initial measures and medications through the hospital course and discharge, based on the latest clinical trials, are outlined in this chapter.

INITIAL MEASURES

Several important initial measures should routinely be performed in the evaluation and treatment of patients with suspected MI.

Twelve-lead Electrocardiography

A 12-lead electrocardiogram (ECG) should be obtained immediately on presentation in the emergency room. Serial ECGs usually should be obtained, especially if the initial ECG shows only nonspecific findings or if the patient's symptoms worsen, as follow-up ECGs may demonstrate new ST-segment elevation (which would make the patient a candidate for thrombolytic therapy).

Continuous Telemetry Monitoring

The majority of deaths early after the onset of MI are due to the occurrence of arrhythmias, particularly ventricular tachycardia and ventricular fibrillation. Prompt recognition and treatment of these frequently fatal arrhythmias is essential in increasing the patient's chances of surviving MI. Therefore, all patients should be continuously monitored for arrhythmias.

Physical Examination

A directed physical examination can give important clues to the extent of ventricular dysfunction and life-threatening complications resulting from the acute MI. Findings of jugular venous distention, rales, or an S3 gallop suggest significant left ventricular dysfunction. The finding of hypotension, jugular venous distention, and clear lung fields suggests right ventricular infarction. The finding of a new holosystolic murmur should raise concerns about either acute mitral regurgitation due to papillary muscle infarction and rupture or the development of a ventricular septal defect. Both papillary muscle rupture with acute mitral regurgitation and ventricular septal defect are associated with extremely high mortality rates and usually require prompt surgical repair.

Supplemental Oxygen

Although it has never been demonstrated that oxygen administration reduces morbidity or mortality, the administration of nasal cannula oxygen (usually at 2 L/min) has become standard practice. In patients in whom initial arterial oxygen saturation (as measured by finger pulse-oximetry) is less than 90%, supplemental oxygen should be titrated to maintain arterial oxygen saturation to levels greater than 90%.

◯ CLINICAL PEARLS ◯

Arterial punctures to obtain arterial blood gases should generally *not* be performed to assess oxygenation status, as the arterial puncture represents a potential source of bleeding in patients who receive thrombolytic therapy.

Sublingual Nitroglycerin

At least one, and usually up to three, sublingual nitroglycerin tablets or sprays should be administered to patients with suspected MI. Because coronary vasoconstriction or vasospasm may contribute to decreased myocardial blood flow, administration of nitroglycerin, a potent coronary arterial dilator, may occasionally significantly ameliorate myocardial ischemia. Sublingual nitroglycerin tablets should be administered with great caution, if at all, in patients with suspected right ventricular infarction, as the resulting venodilation and decrease in right ventricular preload can precipitate severe hypotension. The most commonly used dose of nitroglycerin tablets is the 1:150 (400 µg) tablet.

Analgesia

The pain associated with acute MI leads to increased sympathetic nervous system activity, increasing heart rate, blood pressure, and cardiac contractility. All these effects adversely impact on myocardial oxygen demand. Increased sympathetic activity also may increase the risk of ventricular arrhythmias. Therefore, control of pain is important not only for patient comfort *per se* but also contributes to efforts to minimize the extent of myocardial damage and potential for adverse events. Analgesia usually is achieved by the serial intravenous administration of 2 to 4 mg of morphine intravenously every 5 minutes. Physicians' concerns about potential side effects of morphine including respiratory depression and hypotension frequently result in undertreatment of patients. It should be noted that these side effects occur only rarely, and thus concerns about them should, in general, not interfere with attempts at providing adequate patient analgesia.

WHO TO TREAT WITH LIDOCAINE

In the past, intravenous lidocaine drips frequently were begun prophylactically in all patients with acute MI to decrease the incidence of ventricular fibrillation. A meta-analysis of studies on the use of lidocaine found that although such prophylactic use did decrease the frequency of ventricular fibrillation, the use of prophylactic lidocaine was associated with a trend toward overall *increased* mortality, likely due to fatal bradyarrhythmias and asystole. Therefore, prophylactic lidocaine administration is not recommended in patients with acute MI.

Patients with frequent or sustained ventricular arrhythmias who are relatively clinically stable can be first treated with one or more loading boluses of lidocaine. Once these patients are loaded with lidocaine, a maintenance infusion should be begun.

The initial bolus or loading dose of lidocaine is 1.0 to 1.5 mg/kg intravenously. If necessary, further loading boluses of 0.5 to 0.75 mg/kg can be administered every 5 to 10 minutes up to a total lidocaine dose of 3 mg/kg. Maintenance infusions are usually 2 to 4 mg/min (most commonly 2 mg/min).

◆ CLINICAL PEARLS ◆

In patients who metabolize lidocaine slowly (such as elderly patients, patients with congestive heart failure, and patients with liver disease), the maintenance infusion rate should be lower, to prevent lidocaine toxicity.

MEDICATIONS THAT SHOULD BE CONSIDERED WHEN THE PATIENT FIRST PRESENTS WITH MYOCARDIAL INFARCTION

In patients who present with acute MI, five medications, discussed here and listed in Table 7.1, should be considered in the patient's initial treatment.

Aspirin

Administration of aspirin to patients with acute MI has been shown to decrease mortality by 23%, and this beneficial effect has been shown to be additive with that of thrombolytic therapy. Therefore, treatment with aspirin is now recommended in *virtually all patients* with suspected MI.

Table 7.1. *Five medications that should always be considered in the initial treatment of patients with myocardial infarction*

1. Aspirin
   - 160 mg (two baby aspirin) chewed, then
   - Begin 160–325 mg (usually one 325-mg enteric-coated aspirin) daily.
2. Heparin
   - In patients not treated with thrombolytic therapy: 80 U/kg IV bolus then 18 U/kg/h infusion
   - In patients treated with t-PA 70 U/kg IV bolus then 15 U/kg/h infusion; in patients treated with r-PA: 5000 U IV bolus then initial infusion of 1000 U/h
   - In patients treated with streptokinase: Routine use no longer recommended. If to be given, check PTT 4 h after streptokinase administration. Begin heparin at 1000 U/h (no initial bolus) when PTT <2x control
3. Beta blockers
   - Metoprolol 5 mg IV every 5 min for three doses as tolerated by heart rate and blood pressure
   - Begin metoprolol 50 mg p.o. b.i.d. quickly titrated up to 100 mg p.o. b.i.d. as tolerated
4. Nitroglycerin (intravenous)
   - Initial infusion at 10–20 μg/min, then
   - Titrate dose upward in 10–20 μg/min increments every 5–10 min as clinically indicated and as tolerated by blood pressure
5. Thrombolytic therapy
   - t-PA: 15 mg IV bolus, then 50 mg IV over 30 min, then 35 mg IV over 1 h
   - r-PA: 10mg IV bolus followed by a second 10-mg IV bolus 30 min later
   - Streptokinase: 1.5 million U over 1 h

The only patients who should not be treated with aspirin are those with *true aspirin allergies*. It is important to note that many patients who initially state that they were told that they were allergic to aspirin merely had a mild adverse reaction to it (such as minor stomach upset). It is important to question carefully those patients who say they are "allergic" to aspirin, as the benefit of administering aspirin almost always will outweigh any risk of any minor adverse reaction to aspirin. In patients in whom there is concern about the gastrointestinal effects of aspirin (such as those with active peptic ulcer disease), aspirin can be administered via a rectal suppository. Consider treating patients with true aspirin allergies with clopidogrel (Plavix).

Patients with suspected acute MI should be treated immediately with 160 to 325 mg of aspirin (two baby aspirins or one adult aspirin). The aspirin should be *chewed* to quicken absorption. After initial treatment, 160 to 325 mg of aspirin (most commonly one 325-mg enteric-coated tablet) should be administered daily.

Heparin

In general, all patients not treated with thrombolytic therapy, except those in whom there is a strong contraindication (due primarily to the risk of bleeding), should be treated with heparin. Particularly for those patients at high risk of systemic emboli (large or anterior MI, atrial fibrillation, previous embolus, or known left ventricular thrombus), heparin should be administered intravenously. A weight-adjusted dosing schedule of 80 U/kg bolus then 18 U/kg/h intravenous infusion [later adjusted to partial thromboplastin time (PTT) results] is recommended. Subcutaneous heparin (7,500 U b.i.d.) can be considered in patients at low risk for embolization.

Two recent studies suggest that in patients with non–Q-wave myocardial infarction, treatment with the low molecular weight heparin enoxaparin (Lovenox) reduces adverse outcomes to a greater extent than from treatment with unfractionated heparin. Therefore, the practitioner should consider treating patients with NQMI with enoxaparin 1mg s.c. q12h.

✦ CLINICAL PEARLS ✦

The risk of heparin-induced thrombocytopenia is approximately 3% and has been associated, paradoxically, with a substantial risk of prothrombotic events. Therefore, patients treated with heparin should have daily platelet counts. In those patients in whom platelet count drops below 100,000, a diagnosis of heparin-induced thrombocytopenia should be considered and investigated.

In patients treated with tissue plasminogen activator (t-PA) or r-PA, intravenous unfractionated heparin should be begun at the time of thrombolytic administration. Because high-dose heparin treatment and high PTT levels have been associated with an increased risk of intracranial bleeding, a lower dosing regimen is recommended. Patients treated with t-PA should be treated with a 70 U/kg bolus and then begun on an intravenous infusion of 15 U/kg/h. Patients treated with r-PA should be administered a 5,000-U bolus followed by a continuous infusion at an initial rate of 1,000 U/h. The heparin infusion should be adjusted to maintain a PTT of 1.5 to 2.0 times control (50 to 75 seconds).

Most patients who are treated with t-PA or r-PA should be treated with heparin for approximately 48 hours. Longer treatment periods should be considered in those at high risk of embolization.

Beta Blockers

Patients with MI, particularly those with ST-segment elevation, who present within 12 hours of symptom onset or continue to have anginal chest pain, and do not have contraindications to beta-blocker treatment, should be treated initially with intravenous beta blockers. One suggested regimen is metoprolol (Lopressor) 5 mg intravenously q5min for three doses, assessing for hemodynamic and electrocardiographic stability after each intravenous dose.

Patients who are initially treated with intravenous beta blockers, as well as most other patients with MI, should then be treated with oral beta blockers. One regimen is to begin with metoprolol 50 mg by mouth b.i.d. for the first day, then quickly titrate the dose up to 100 m.g. b.i.d.

Nitroglycerin

Intravenous nitroglycerin should definitely be used in patients with large anterior MI, congestive heart failure, hypertension, and/or persistent ischemia, and its use should be considered in all patients with acute MI. It should be avoided in patients with hypotension and/or right ventricular infarction. Intravenous nitroglycerin should be begun at a rate of 10 to 20 µg/min. This rate should be titrated upward in 10 to 20 µg/min increments every 5 to 10 minutes as tolerated by blood pressure. Titration endpoints should include relief of pain and lowering of systolic blood pressure by 10% in normotensive patients and by 30% in hypertensive patients (but not below a systolic blood pressure of 90 mm Hg). Intravenous nitroglycerin should be maintained for 24 to 48 hours and then titrated to off if the patient experiences no further ischemia. At present, there is no evidence that long-acting oral nitrates should be started once the intravenous nitroglycerin is tapered off.

◆ CLINICAL PEARLS ◆

Several reports suggest that intravenous nitroglycerin may interfere with the anticoagulant effects of heparin. Therefore, care givers should be aware that patients treated with both agents may require higher doses of heparin and should have their PTT levels monitored carefully. Additionally, caregivers should be aware that in those patients treated with both agents and in whom the PTT is in the therapeutic range, discontinuation of nitroglycerin and continued heparin treatment at the same dose may, at least theoretically, increase the risk of bleeding, and thus warrant renewed careful monitoring of the PTT.

Thrombolytic Agents

Multiple large randomized trials have now conclusively demonstrated that administration of thrombolytic agents to select patients with acute MI significantly decreased mortality. The benefits are greatest in those with electrocardiographic findings of a left bundle branch block (LBBB) that is not known to be old (i.e., the LBBB has not been noted on a previous ECG and therefore is presumed to be due to the MI) and those with anterior ST-segment elevation. Patients with inferior or lateral ST elevations derive modest but real benefit from thrombolytic treatment. Patients with nonspecific electrocardiographic changes do not derive any benefit from thrombolytic treatment and those with ST-segment depression who are treated with thrombolytics tend to do worse when compared to no thrombolytic treatment.

Patients who are treated quickly (less than 6 hours) after the onset of symptoms derive the greatest benefit from thrombolytic treatment. However, several studies suggest that patients treated even 7 to 12 hours after symptom onset, particularly if they have a large MI or are continuing to have angina, still derive benefit from thrombolytic therapy.

Based on these findings, it is recommended that patients with electrocardiographic findings of ≥1-mm ST-segment elevation in two or more contiguous leads or LBBB not known to be old who present within 6 to 12 hours of symptom onset should be treated with thrombolytic therapy.

As would be expected, the major complication of thrombolytic administration is bleeding. Absolute and relative contraindications to thrombolytic therapy are listed in Table 7.2.

Trials comparing different thrombolytic agents have detected either no, or only modest, overall differences among these agents with regard to efficacy and side effects, and the nuances of which agent to consider in which patient are both too complex to discuss in this book and not as clinically important as the actual decision to administer a thrombolytic agent to a

Table 7.2. *Absolute and relative contraindications for thrombolytic use in patients with acute myocardial infarction*

Absolute contraindications
• Previous hemorrhagic stroke at any time or thromboembolic stroke within 1 yr
• Known intracranial neoplasm
• Active internal bleeding (not menses)
• Suspected aortic dissection

Relative contraindications
• Severe hypertension ($>^{180}/_{110}$) or history of severe hypertension
• Recent trauma or surgery (with 2–4 wk) or prolonged cardiopulmonary resuscitation (>10 min)
• Recent internal bleeding (within 2–4 wk) or active peptic ulcer
• Bleeding diathesis or current use of warfarin with INR >2–3
• Pregnancy

patient. Tissue plasminogen activator is administered as an initial 15-mg bolus followed by 0.75 mg/kg (not to exceed 50 mg) administered over 30 minutes followed by 0.50 mg/kg (not to exceed 35 mg) administered over 1 hour (total dose 100 mg in most patients). r-PA (Retavase) is administered as an initial 10-mg bolus followed 30 minutes later by a second 10-mg bolus. Streptokinase is administered as 1.5 million units over 1 hour.

PLATELET IIB/IIIA RECEPTOR INHIBITORS

Who to Consider for Treatment

Recent studies have demonstrated that the use of medications that block the platelet IIb/IIIa receptor and inhibit platelet aggregation may provide benefit in reduction of adverse events (death, MI, recurrent ischemia) beyond that obtained with aspirin and unfractionated heparin alone in patients with acute coronary syndromes, including those with non–Q-wave MI. These agents may be considered in patients who present with ST-segment depression or T-wave inversions that are likely due to ischemia, and in patients with positive troponin or creatine kinase-MB levels. If used, platelet IIb/IIIa inhibitors should be utilized in addition to standard therapy, including aspirin, heparin, and antianginal agents. These agents should not be utilized in patients who present with ST-segment elevation and who are to be treated with thrombolytic therapy.

Available Agents

At the time of this writing, approved regimens include the following:

Eptifibatide (Integrilin): Administer 180 µg/kg bolus then 2 µg/kg/min continuous infusion for up to 72 hours (*Note:* dose is in micrograms, not milligrams). Treat with aspirin and intravenous heparin (with target PTT 50 to 75 seconds). It should not be used in patients with creatinine ≥2.0 mg/dL.

Tirofiban (Aggrastat): Administer initial 0.4 µg/kg/min intravenously for 30 minutes then continuous intravenous infusion at 0.1 µg/kg/min (*Note:* dose is in micrograms, not milligrams). Treat with aspirin and intravenous heparin (with target PTT approximately two times control). Patients with severely impaired renal function should receive half the usual initial loading dose and half the usual continuous infusion rate. Check platelet count within 6 hours following administrations of loading infusion and daily thereafter (monitor for rare thrombocytopenia).

A third agent, *abciximab (ReoPro),* currently is undergoing study in patients with acute coronary syndromes.

Contraindications to Use

Contraindications to the use of IIb/IIIa inhibitors vary slightly between products, but generally include those factors that predispose to increased bleeding risks, including prior intracranial hemorrhage or history of recent stroke of any kind, recent or ongoing bleeding, recent major surgery or trauma, severe hypertension, or below normal platelet count (consult the manufacturer's package monogram before using for a full listing of contraindications).

CARE OF THE PATIENT OVER THE FIRST SEVERAL DAYS

During the first several days of the patient's stay in the cardiac care unit, the patient is observed carefully for recurrent chest pain and for the development of arrhythmias or congestive heart failure. Several medication adjustments and other measures should be considered during this time. These are discussed here and summarized in Table 7.3.

Tapering and Discontinuation of Intravenous Medications

If the patient remains angina-free for 1 to 2 days, intravenous nitroglycerin can be tapered to off and the patient can be switched to nitropaste (1 to 2 in. applied every 6 hours). As noted previously, in patients with uncomplicated MIs, after several days intravenous heparin can be discontinued. In patients who were begun on lidocaine for ventricular arrhythmias at the time of the acute MI but have since had no further arrhythmias, lidocaine treatment usually is tapered to off.

Table 7.3. *Management considerations over the first several days in patients with myocardial infarction*

---

1. Tapering and discontinuing intravenous medications
   - In patients without recurrent chest pain, after 1–2 d taper IV nitroglycerin to off; can begin nitropaste ("NTP") 1–2 inches q6h
   - In patient with uncomplicated myocardial infarction and no recurrent chest pain, after 2 d discontinue i.v. heparin
   - In patients begun on lidocaine but with no further arrhythmias, after several days can taper lidocaine to off
2. In patients with uncomplicated initial hospital course, after 2 d can transfer to intermediate care or step-down unit
3. In patients with uncomplicated initial hospital course, increase activities and ambulation
4. Consider obtaining cardiac echocardiogram
5. ACE inhibitors
   - Definitely start ACE inhibitors in patients with (i) large anterior myocardial infarction; (ii) ejection fraction <40%; and/or (iii) congestive heart failure
   - Consider starting ACE inhibitors in all patients without myocardial infarction (without contraindications)
   - Start treatment 1 to several days after myocardial infarction
   - Start dose low but titrate up quickly to higher-end doses

---

ACE, angiotensin-converting enzyme.

Increasing Activities

In patients who remain angina-free and are not in congestive heart failure, activity can be increased gradually over several days, first allowing the patient to get out of bed, then to ambulate within the patient's room, and then in the hallways.

Cardiac Echocardiography

Although it is not considered "mandatory" to obtain a cardiac echocardiogram in the initial care of the patient with acute MI, information derived from the echocardiogram, particularly the patient's left ventricular ejection fraction and ventricular wall-motion abnormalities, are helpful in selecting medications and guiding later management.

Angiotensin-converting Enzyme Inhibitors

In patients who have suffered acute MI, studies have demonstrated that early treatment with angiotensin-converting enzyme (ACE) inhibitors has been shown to reduce left ventricular dysfunction, reduce left ventricular dilation, and slow progression to congestive heart failure and decrease mortality. Patients who derive the most benefit from early treatment with

ACE inhibitors and clearly should be treated with these agents include patients with:

- Large anterior MI
- Depressed ejection fraction (less than 40%)
- Congestive heart failure.

Angiotensin-converting enzyme inhibitors appear to provide at least some modest benefit in all patients with acute MI and, therefore, can be considered in all patients with acute MI.

An oral ACE inhibitor should be started within 1 to several days after acute MI. Although the starting dose should be low (as some people manifest significant drops in blood pressure with ACE-inhibitor therapy), *the dose should quickly be titrated to high doses* as tolerated by blood pressure and kidney function. Experts have repeatedly lamented the fact that most people are treated with doses much lower than those used in clinical trials (for example, the *average* dose of captopril in the SAVE trial was 50 mg t.i.d.). Starting and target doses for the available ACE inhibitors are summarized in Chapter 1. Treatment with ACE inhibitors should be continued for 4 to 6 weeks.

During treatment, patients should be observed for hypotension, *significant* impairment of renal function such as hyperkalemia or oliguria *(modest rises in blood urea nitrogen and/or creatinine should not, in itself, be reason to discontinue ACE inhibitor therapy),* and angioedema.

Bed Management

Patients who remain angina-free, who are not in congestive heart failure, and who have not had significant arrhythmias can be transferred from the CCU to an intermediate care or "step-down" unit after 48 hours in the Coronary Care Unit (CCU). Most practitioners continue telemetry monitoring during this period.

PREDISCHARGE PLANNING

Anticoagulation

In patients who are found on cardiac echocardiogram to have a large anterior MI with an akinetic (not moving) anterior wall and/or an akinetic or dyskinetic (moving paradoxically) apex, warfarin (Coumadin) usually is prescribed for 3 to 6 months to decrease the chances of a thrombus forming (and embolizing) (Table 7.4). Patients found on echocardiogram to be at risk for thrombus formation should be continued on heparin in the hospital until a therapeutic international normalized ratio of 2 to 3 is achieved with warfarin treatment.

Table 7.4. *Predischarge planning considerations*

1. Anticoagulate with warfarin 3–6 m in those with large anterior myocardial infarction (target INR = 2–3)
2. Predischarge stress test 5–7 d after admission
   - Order a "submaximal" or "modified" exercise test in most patients
   - Order a nuclear or echo imaging study in those with (i) significant ST-segment abnormalities; (ii) those taking digoxin; and (iii) those with left bundle branch block on electrocardiogram
3. Consider cardiac catheterization in patients with
   - Recurrent angina
   - Positive predischarge stress test
   - Patients who present with ischemic pulmonary edema
   - Patients with moderately or severely depressed ejection fraction who are suspected of having multivessel coronary artery disease

Exercise and Pharmacologic Stress Testing

In patients who remain stable during their hospital course, a predischarge exercise test should be obtained 5 to 7 days after initial hospital admission (Fig. 7.1). Most physicians will order a modified or submaximal exercise test (in which the patient is only exercised for a certain amount of time or until the heart rate reaches 70% of the maximum predicted heart rate). In those patients who have significant baseline ST-segment abnormalities, are on digoxin, or have a left bundle branch block, an imaging study (usually a nuclear imaging or echocardiographic study) should be considered, because these three factors make reliable interpretation of electrocardiographic changes during the stress test impossible. In patients who cannot exercise (such as those with severe claudication or those with amputations), a persantine or adenosine test should be ordered in the nuclear medicine department or through the cardiac echocardiography laboratory.

Who to Refer for Cardiac Catheterization

Practice patterns differ in different parts of the country and even among physicians as to which patients with MI should undergo cardiac catheterization (Fig. 7.1). There are, however, several indications for cardiac catheterization that are almost universally agreed on. These indications are as follows:

- Recurrent angina during the hospital course
- Inducible angina and/or signs of ischemia during the predischarge stress test

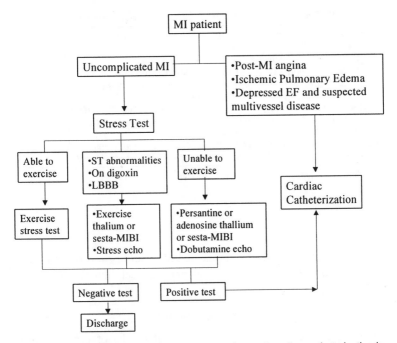

FIG. 7.1. Considerations regarding exercise testing and cardiac catheterization in hospitalized patients with myocardial infarction.

- Patients who present with ischemic pulmonary edema (because these patients have a poorer long-term prognosis and a high incidence of three vessel or left main coronary artery disease)
- Patients with moderately or severely depressed ejection fractions (on cardiac echocardiogram) in whom multivessel coronary artery disease is suspected to be the etiology.

POSTDISCHARGE MANAGEMENT AND SECONDARY PREVENTION

Activities

Whereas in the past patients who suffered MI often were confined to bed rest for weeks, more recently there has been a change in thinking, with patients encouraged to resume physical activities and work (Table 7.5). Daily walking can be begun immediately, and sexual activity can be resumed 1 week to 10 days after discharge. Although there are little firm data to support specific recommendations on driving and return to work,

Table 7.5. *Postdischarge considerations and secondary prevention*

1. Regarding activities, inform the patient that he or she can
   - Resume daily walking immediately
   - Resume sexual activities 7–10 d after discharge
   - Resume driving after about 1 wk if uncomplicated myocardial infarction
   - Return to work after about 2 wk if uncomplicated myocardial infarction
2. Strongly encourage smoking cessation
3. Treat with aspirin indefinitely (usually one 325-mg enteric-coated tablet daily)
4. Treat with beta blockers (unless strong contraindications) indefinitely (one regimen is metoprolol 100 mg p.o. b.i.d.)
5. Check total and low-density lipoprotein cholesterol levels, initiate dietary modification, and, if lipids elevated, treat with a HMG-coA reductase inhibitor.

HMG-CoA, hydroxymethylglutaryl coenzyme A.

in general patients with uncomplicated MIs can begin driving 1 week after discharge and can return to work about 2 weeks after discharge.

Smoking Cessation

Smoking cessation dramatically reduces the risks of cardiovascular events, and all patients should be instructed in the strongest possible terms to stop smoking.

Medications

Treatment of MI survivors with aspirin has been shown in multiple studies to decrease recurrent vascular events and vascular mortality. Although different doses of aspirin were used in these studies, most physicians in the United States now prescribe one 325-mg enteric-coated aspirin daily indefinitely. Patients allergic to or intolerant of aspirin should be treated with clopidogrel (Plavix) 75 mg q.d. Several studies have demonstrated that treatment with beta blockers also decreases subsequent mortality. All patients without strong contraindications to beta blockers should be treated indefinitely with beta blockers. One reasonable regimen is metoprolol 100 mg by mouth b.i.d.

Cholesterol Reduction

Several studies have now established that treatment of elevated total and/or low-density lipoprotein (LDL) cholesterol reduces subsequent mortality. Based on these studies, most cardiologists will now treat patients with total cholesterols greater than 240 mg/dL and/or with LDL cholesterol levels greater than 100–130 mg/dL on a 3-hydroxy-3-methyl-glutaryl coenzyme A reductase inhibitor ("statin"), with the goal of lowering LDL cholesterol to less than 100 mg/dL. All patients should also undergo dietary modification. Suggested regimens and the treatment of hypercholesterolemia are discussed further in Chapter 9.

◖ CLINICAL PEARLS ◗

Cholesterol levels fall within 24 hours of hospital admission. Therefore, if cholesterol levels are not checked within this time frame and are checked later during the hospitalization and found not to be elevated, they should be rechecked 6 to 12 weeks after discharge.

SUMMARY

Care of the patient with MI can be divided into initial measures, a consideration of five medications to use in the immediate treatment of the patient, care of the patient over the first several days, predischarge planning, and postdischarge management. Appropriate utilization of medications during these periods can allow the primary care provider to significantly and positively impact his or her patient's care and prognosis.

8

Evaluation and Treatment of the Patient with Hypertension

Glenn N. Levine

*Baylor College of Medicine, Cardiac Catheterization Laboratory,
Houston V. A. Medical Center, Houston, Texas 77030*

More than 50 million Americans have hypertension. Untreated or inadequately treated hypertension can contribute to coronary artery disease, congestive heart failure, stroke, and end-stage renal disease. Although studies suggest that recognition and treatment of hypertension may significantly reduce the morbidity associated with this condition, only about one fourth of those with hypertension are believed to be adequately treated.

In this chapter, the evaluation of the patient found to have elevated blood pressure and the latest recommendations on the treatment of hypertension are discussed. Recommendations from the *Sixth Report of the Joint National Committee on Prevention, Detection, Evaluation, and Treatment of High Blood Pressure (JNC-VI)*, as well as from the *National High Blood Pressure Education Program Working Group Report on Hypertension in the Elderly* and the *World Health Organization Technical Report on Hypertension Control* are incorporated into evaluation and management recommendations.

An overall algorithm for the evaluation of the patient with measured elevated blood pressure and for the evaluation and management of patients diagnosed with hypertension is provided in Fig. 8.1.

INITIAL TRIAGING OF THE PATIENT WITH A MEASURED ELEVATED BLOOD PRESSURE

The diagnosis of hypertension should never be based on one blood pressure reading alone. For most patients (except those with hypertensive

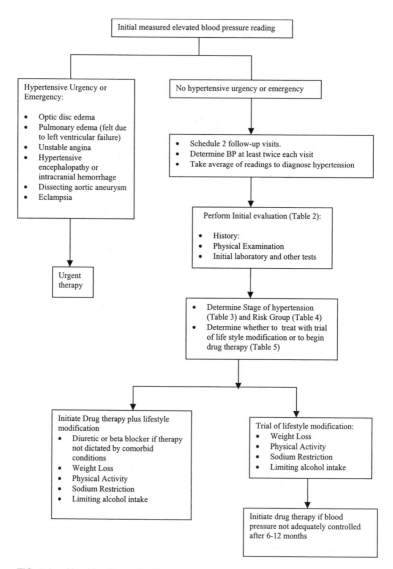

FIG. 8.1. Algorithm for evaluation and management of patients with hypertension.

urgency or hypertensive crisis, discussed in the following paragraph), two follow-up visits, spaced several weeks apart, should be scheduled for further assessment of the patient's blood pressure. At each of these two visits, two blood pressure readings, at least several minutes apart, should be taken. If these two readings differ by more than 5 mm Hg, a third reading

TABLE 8.1. *Measuring blood pressure in the office setting*

- Patients should be seated with the arms supported at heart level.
- Patients should not smoke or ingest caffeine for the 30 minutes prior to blood pressure measurement.
- Patients should be seated for at least 5 minutes before blood pressure is measured.
- The bladder of the blood pressure cuff should encircle at least 80% of the arm (otherwise, blood pressure readings may be falsely elevated). Use a large (or even thigh) cuff in those with large arms.
- Two or more readings at least 2 minutes apart should be obtained.

should be obtained and the three measurements averaged. The proper steps in measuring blood pressure in the office setting are outlined in Table 8.1.

✪ CLINICAL PEARLS ✪

The bladder of the blood pressure cuff should encircle at least 80% of the arm. Otherwise, blood pressure readings may be falsely elevated. Use a large cuff (or even a thigh cuff) with patients who have large arms.

Patients with markedly elevated blood pressures and signs or symptoms of hypertensive urgency or hypertensive emergency should receive acute antihypertensive treatment. Signs and symptoms include:

Optic disc edema
Pulmonary edema (thought to result from left ventricular failure)
Unstable angina
Hypertensive encephalopathy or intracranial hemorrhage
Dissecting aortic aneurysm
Eclampsia.

In these patients, the blood pressure should be initially lowered by 25% over the first several hours. It then should be lowered further over 2 to 6 hours to a level of $160/100$ mm Hg. The practitioner should take care to reduce blood pressure gradually; sharp reductions can lead to cerebral hypoperfusion.

DIAGNOSIS AND EVALUATION OF THE HYPERTENSIVE PATIENT

Once the patient with an initially measured elevated blood pressure has had two follow-up visits, the average of two or more blood pressure readings taken in the course of the two follow-up evaluations should be calculated. Patients with an average systolic blood pressure greater than 140 mm Hg, an average diastolic blood pressure greater than 90 mm Hg, or both, are considered to have hypertension.

Once the diagnosis of hypertension is established, a comprehensive evaluation of the patient should be performed. This can be done during the second follow-up visit. The comprehensive evaluation should achieve three goals:

1. Assessment for target organ damage and cardiovascular disease
2. Identification of other cardiovascular risk factors (which will help determine the choice of therapy)
3. Identification of possible secondary causes of hypertension.

History

The practitioner should question the patient regarding the known presence of—or symptoms suggestive of—coronary artery disease, congestive heart failure, and cerebrovascular or peripheral vascular disease; the presence of other cardiac risk factors; lifestyle factors (diet, sodium intake, alcohol intake, tobacco use, leisure-time physical activity, caffeine use); and medication use (both prescription and over-the-counter drugs).

Physical Examination

The physical examination should include measurement of blood pressure in both arms (the higher reading between the two arms should be used); fundoscopic examination; neck examination for carotid bruits or enlarged thyroid; cardiac examination for heaves, murmurs, or extra heart sounds; abdominal examination for bruits, masses, enlarged kidneys, or aortic aneurysm; and examination of the extremities for femoral bruits or diminished distal pulses.

Laboratory Tests and Other Diagnostic Tests

The following blood tests should be performed on all patients diagnosed with hypertension:

- Hematocrit
- Blood chemistries (particularly creatinine, potassium, sodium, fasting glucose, and cholesterol)
- Urinalysis
- Electrocardiogram.

Additional studies to consider in the evaluation of select patients with hypertension include blood calcium, low-density lipoprotein cholesterol,

---

TABLE 8.2. *Checklist for initial evaluation of patients with hypertension*

History
   ? Coronary artery disease, congestive heart failure, stroke, or peripheral vascular disease
   ? Other cardiac risk factors
   ? Lifestyle factors (diet, sodium and alcohol intake, smoking, leisure-time physical activity, caffeine use)
   ? Medication use (prescription and over the counter)

Physical examination
   • Blood pressures in both arms
   • Fundoscopic exam
   ? Carotid bruits or thyroid mass
   ? Cardiac heaves, murmurs, or extra heart sounds
   ? Abdominal bruits, masses, enlarged kidneys, or aortic aneurysm
   ? Femoral bruits or diminished distal pulses

Strongly recommended initial laboratory and other tests on all patients
   • Hematocrit
   • Blood chemistries (creatinine, potassium, sodium, fasting glucose, and cholesterol)
   • Urinalysis
   • Electrocardiogram

Other tests to consider
   • Calcium
   • Low-density lipoprotein cholesterol
   • Thyroid-stimulating hormone
   • Uric acid
   • 24-hour urinary protein
   • Creatinine clearance

---

thyroid-stimulating hormone, uric acid, 24-hour urinary protein, and creatinine clearance. Table 8.2 provides a checklist for the evaluation of hypertensive patients.

HOW TO DETERMINE INITIAL TREATMENT FOR THE PATIENT WITH HYPERTENSION

Once diagnosis and evaluation have been completed, the next step in treating the patient with hypertension is to determine the initial treatment strategy. This initial treatment strategy should be based on both the stage of hypertension and the JNC-VI risk group, as discussed in the following paragraphs.

Stages of Hypertension

Based on average blood pressure, the patient's stage of hypertension should be classified according to *JNC-VI* guidelines. The *JNC-VI* classes

Table 8.3. *JNC-VI classification of blood pressure and the stages of hypertension*

Category	Systolic blood pressure (mmHg)		Diastolic blood pressure (mmHg)
Optimal	<120	and	<80
Normal	<130	and	<85
High-normal	130–139	or	85–89
Hypertension			
Stage 1	140–159	or	90–99
Stage 2	160–179	or	100–109
Stage 3	180	or	110

of blood pressure and stages of hypertension are shown in Table 8.3. When systolic and diastolic readings fall into different stages, the higher stage should be used to categorize the degree of hypertension.

Risk Group Stratification

Patients also should be categorized as to the "risk group" they fall into. The *JNC-VI* criteria for risk groups A, B, and C are provided in Table 8.4.

Initial Treatment Strategies

The most important early treatment decision is whether to try a period of lifestyle modification or proceed directly to drug therapy (along with lifestyle modification). The suggested initial treatment strategy, based on the patient's stage of hypertension and risk group, is presented in Table 8.5.

Stage 1 Hypertension ($^{140-159}/_{85-89}$ mm Hg)

Patients with stage 1 hypertension and no more than one coronary risk factor (other than diabetes) should be treated with a trial of lifestyle modification (discussed later) for 6 to 12 months. If, after this period, blood pressure remains elevated, then antihypertensive pharmacotherapy should be initiated. Patients with stage 1 hypertension and diabetes, target organ damage, or clinical cardiovascular disease should be started on drug therapy (as well as lifestyle modification).

Stage 2 and Stage 3 Hypertension ($\geq^{160}/_{100}$ mm Hg)

All patients determined to have stage 2 or stage 3 hypertension should be started on drug therapy (as well as lifestyle modification).

TABLE. 8.4. *JNC-VI classifications of risk of cardiovascular disease*

Risk group A
 • No other major cardiac risk factors[a]
 • No target organ damage or clinical cardiovascular disease[b]
Risk group B
 • One major cardiac risk factor other than diabetes
 • No target organ damage or clinical cardiovascular disease[b]
Risk group C
 • Presence of diabetes (with or without other cardiac risk factors)
                           and/or
 • Presence of target organ damage and/or clinical cardiovascular disease

 [a] Major risk factors as defined for the purposes of the *Sixth Report of the Joint National Committee on Prevention, Detection, Evaluation, and Treatment of High Blood Pressure* (*JNC*) classification system include smoking, dyslipidemia, diabetes mellitus, men age greater than 60 yr or postmenopausal women, and family history of cardiovascular disease (women less than 65 yr or men less than 55 yr).
 [b] Target organ damage and/or clinical cardiovascular disease as defined for the purposes of the *JNC* classification system include heart disease (left ventricular hypertrophy, angina, prior myocardial infarction, prior coronary revascularization, or heart failure), stroke or transient ischemic attack, nephropathy, peripheral arterial disease, or retinopathy.
 (Adapted from the Sixth Report of the Joint National Committee on Prevention, Detection, Evaluation, and Treatment of High Blood Pressure. *Arch Intern Med* 1997.)

TARGET BLOOD PRESSURES

The goal of both nonpharmacologic and pharmacologic therapy in most patients should be to lower blood pressure to less than $140/90$ mm Hg. Patients with diabetes mellitus and those with renal parenchymal disease with proteinuria should have their blood pressure lowered to less than $130/85$ mm Hg. In patients with established atherosclerotic disease, blood pressure should be lowered to at least $140/90$ mm Hg; lowering blood pressure to a target level of $130/85$ mm Hg may be desirable, provided this lowering of perfusion pressures has no adverse effects on the patient (e.g., lightheadedness). In young and middle-aged patients, even lower target blood pressures of $120/80$ to $130/80$ mm Hg are recommended by the World Health Organization.

TREATING PATIENTS WITH ISOLATED SYSTOLIC HYPERTENSION

Isolated systolic hypertension (an elevated systolic blood pressure in the setting of a normal diastolic blood pressure) is a common finding in elderly patients. As treatment of isolated systolic hypertension has been shown to decrease vascular morbidity, patients with this condition should be treated like other patients with hypertension, with the goal of lowering

Table 8.5. *JNC-VI recommendations for initial treatment of patients with high-normal blood pressure and frank hypertension*

Blood pressure stage (mm Hg)	Risk group A (no coronary risk factors, no target organ disease/ clinical cardiovascular disease)	Risk group B (one coronary risk factor except diabetes, no target organ disease/ clinical cardiovascular disease)	Risk group C (target organ disease/ clinical cardiovascular disease and/or diabetes)
High-normal (130–139/85–89)	Lifestyle modification	Lifestyle modification	Drug therapy
Stage 1 (140–159/90–99)	Lifestyle modification (up to 12 mo)[a]	Life style modification (up to 6 mo) if only one CRF[a]	Consider drug therapy if more than one CRF Drug therapy
Stage 2 and 3 (160/100)	Drug therapy	Drug therapy	Drug therapy

[a] If target blood pressure not achieved after this period, begin pharmacologic therapy.
CRF, cardiac risk factor.
(Adapted from the Sixth Report of the Joint National Committee on Prevention, Detection, Evaluation, and Treatment of High Blood Pressure. *Arch Intern Med* 1997.)

systolic blood pressure to less than 140 mm Hg. In those patients with marked systolic hypertension, an interim goal of lowering systolic blood pressure to less than 160 mm Hg may be prudent, to avoid lowering cerebral perfusion pressure too quickly.

LIFESTYLE MODIFICATIONS

For some patients, lifestyle modifications may be sufficient to achieve target blood pressure goals. Even for those who require pharmacologic therapy, the nonpharmacologic steps discussed in the following paragraphs may reduce the number of medications and number of doses needed to control blood pressure. The following lifestyle modifications should be discussed with all patients.

Weight Loss

All overweight patients should be encouraged to lose weight through a combination of modified caloric intake and increased physical activity. A goal of 10 to 15 lb in many patients is reasonable.

Physical Activity

Patients should be encouraged to engage in moderate aerobic physical activity, such as brisk walks 3 to 5 days a week. Patients with known cardiac disease or symptoms suggestive of coronary artery disease should undergo exercise stress testing before embarking on such an exercise program.

Sodium Restriction

Patients should be instructed to limit daily sodium intake to no more than 2.4 g. As processed foods contain large amounts of sodium, a good first step is to avoid processed foods whenever possible.

Limiting Alcohol Intake

Patients with hypertension should be instructed to limit daily alcohol intake to 1 oz of alcohol (i.e., no more than 24 oz of beer, 10 oz of wine, or 2 oz of 100-proof alcohol).

CHOOSING WHICH PHARMACOLOGIC
AGENT TO PRESCRIBE

In patients without any comorbid conditions for whom a certain type of antihypertensive agent may be preferable to treat the comorbid condition, the first-line antihypertensive agent should be a diuretic or a beta blocker. Long-acting (i.e., once-a-day) preparations are preferable to short-acting agents.

Cost should be considered with patients who must pay for their own medications. Patients who cannot afford the medication are likely to comply poorly with the medication regime. Diuretics (particularly hydrochlorothiazide) and generic preparations may cost less than brand-name agents.

Certain antihypertensive medications should be considered with certain populations and with patients with certain comorbid conditions.

African-American Patients

Because African-Americans may be somewhat less responsive to the antihypertensive effects of angiotensin-converting enzyme (ACE) inhibitors and beta blockers, other agents, such as diuretics and calcium channel blockers, should be initially considered. However, if comorbid conditions, such as congestive heart failure, are present that require medications such as ACE inhibitors and beta blockers, then these agents should be used.

Older Patients

Older patients derive significant benefit from antihypertensive therapy, and they should not be treated less aggressively than younger patients just because they are older. At present, the preferred agents are diuretics and beta blockers. Dihydropyridine calcium blockers are reasonable alternatives. Peripheral vasodilators should be avoided because of the risk of postural hypotension; centrally acting agents create the risk of impaired cognitive function and should be avoided. Smaller starting doses of medications should be used with older patients. The starting dose of hydrochlorothiazide should be no more than 12.5 mg daily.

Patients with Coronary Artery Disease

Beta blockers are good first-choice agents for most patients with concomitant coronary artery disease. Angiotensin-converting enzyme inhibitors are ideal agents in patients with depressed left ventricular ejection fraction. Long-acting calcium channel agents may be reasonable second-line agents in patients with angina. Short-acting calcium channel blockers should not be used.

Patients with Depressed Left Ventricular Ejection Fraction

As discussed in Chapter 1, patients with depressed left ventricular ejection fraction or clinical congestive heart failure resulting from systolic dysfunction benefit from treatment with ACE inhibitors and beta blockers. These agents should be first-line agents in the treatment of patients with hypertension.

Patients with Left Ventricular Hypertrophy

Use of the most common antihypertensive agents may lead to at least some regression of left ventricular hypertrophy. The combination of an ACE inhibitor and a diuretic may be more efficacious than other medications. Direct vasodilators have not been shown to be of benefit in reducing left ventricular hypertrophy.

Patients with Renal Disease

Angiotensin-converting enzyme inhibitors should be considered first-choice therapy for patients with diabetic nephropathy, proteinuria (more than 1 g per 24 hours), or impaired renal function. However, ACE inhibitors must be used with extreme caution, if at all, in patients with creatinine levels 3.0 mg/dL or higher, or in those who have known or suspected renal artery stenoses. Diuretics should be considered as an additional agent in those patients who do not achieve adequate blood pressure control with an ACE inhibitor. In patients with significant proteinuria, the target blood pressure is $130/85$ mm Hg or lower.

Patients with Diabetes

Most commonly used agents are acceptable in the treatment of diabetic patients with hypertension. Angiotensin-converting enzyme inhibitors are preferred with patients who have diabetic nephropathy. Particularly with patients who have coronary artery disease or depressed left ventricular ejection fraction, beta blockers should not be avoided solely because of concerns that they may mask the symptoms of hypoglycemia. Blood pressure in patients with diabetes should be reduced to less than $130/85$ mm Hg.

WHEN TO SCHEDULE FOLLOW-UP VISITS

Initial follow-up after beginning therapy should be within 1 to 2 months in uncomplicated patients.

The patient started on ACE inhibitors should be seen within several weeks to verify that kidney function is not severely impaired (e.g., oliguria, hyperkalemia). The patient started on diuretics should be seen in several weeks to verify that he or she is not becoming hypokalemic. Patients with congestive heart failure who are started on beta blockers should be seen within several weeks to verify that the beta blocker is not worsening the congestive heart failure. Management of these patients is discussed in detail in Chapter 1.

Once blood pressure is adequately controlled, follow-up visits should be scheduled at intervals of 3 to 6 months.

WHAT TO DO WHEN BLOOD PRESSURE IS NOT CONTROLLED WITH ONE AGENT

In patients whose hypertension is not controlled with one antihypertensive agent, there are two options: either add a second agent or discontinue the initial agent and try a new one. In patients who are tolerating the initial agent well, the addition of a diuretic (even at low dose) can potentiate the antihypertensive effects. Thus, if a second agent is to be added, it should be a diuretic unless there are compelling reasons to do otherwise. In patients with significant side effects from the first agent, a different agent should be tried.

Medications and doses used in the treatment of hypertension are listed in Table 8.6.

Table 8.6. *Antihypertensive agents and suggested initial and maximum doses*

Medication (brand name)	Initial dose	Maximum dose
Alpha-adrenergic blockers (peripheral)[a]		
Doxazosin (Cardura)	1 mg q.d.	16 mg q.d.
Terazosin (Hytrin)	1 mg q.d.	20 mg q.d.
Angiotension-converting enzyme inhibitors[b]		
Benazepril (Lotensin)	10 mg q.d.	20 mg b.i.d. or 40 mg q.d.
Captopril (Capoten)	25 mg b.i.d.–t.i.d.	50 mg b.i.d.–t.i.d.
Enalapril (Vasotec)	2.5–5 mg q.d.	20 mg b.i.d. or 40 mg q.d.
Fosinopril (Monopril)	10 mg q.d.	40–80 mg q.d.
Lisinopril (Prinivil, Zestril)	10 mg q.d.	40 mg q.d.
Quinapril (Accupril)	10–20 mg q.d.	40 mg b.i.d. or 80 mg q.d.
Ramipril (Altace)	2.5 mg q.d.	10 mg b.i.d. or 20 mg q.d.
Trandolapril (Mavik)	1–2 mg q.d.	4 mg q.d.
Alpha and beta blockers		
Carvedilol (Coreg)	6.25 mg b.i.d.	25 mg b..id.
Labetolol (Normodyne, Trandate)	100 mg b.i.d.	1200 mg b.i.d.
Angiotensin II receptor blockers (ARB)[b]		
Irbesartan (Avapro)	150 mg q.d.	300 mg q.d.
Losartan (Cozaar)	50 mg q.d.	50 mg b.i.d. or 100 mg q.d.
Valsartan (Diovan)	80 mg q.d.	320 mg q.d.

Continued

Table 8.6. *Continued*

Medication (brand name)	Initial dose	Maximum dose
Beta blockers		
Atenolol (Tenormin)	50 mg q.d.	100 mg q.d.
Bisoprolol (Zebeta)	2.5–50 mg q.d.	20 mg q.d.
Metoprolol		
• Lopressor	50 mg b.i.d.	100–200 mg b.i.d.
• Toprol XL	50–100 mg q.d.	200–400 mg q.d.
Nadolol	40 mg q.d.	320 mg q.d.
Propanolol		
• Inderal	40 mg b.i.d.	120–240 mg b.i.d.
• Inderal LA	80 mg q.d.	240–480 mg q.d.
Timolol (Blocadron)	10 mg b.i.d.	30 mg b.i.d.
Calcium channel blockers		
Amlodipine (Norvasc)	2.3–5 mg q.d.	10 mg q.d.
Diltiazem		
• Cardizem SR	60 mg b.i.d.	180 mg b.i.d.
• Cardizem CD, Dilacor, XR,	120–80 mg q.d.	360 mg q.d.
• Tiazac		
Felodipine (Plendil)	5 mg q.d.	10 mg q.d.
Isradipine		
• DynaCirc	2.5 mg b.i.d.	5 mg b.i.d.
• DynaCirc CR	5 mg q.d.	10 mg q.d.
Nicardipine (Cardene SR)	30 mg b.i.d.	60 mg b.i.d.
Nisoldipine (Sular)	20 mg q.d.	60 mg q.d.
Verapamil		
• Calan SR[c], Isoptin SR[c]	180 mg q.d.	240 mg b.i.d.
• Verelan	120 mg qd	480 mg q.d.
• Covera HS	180 mg hs	480 mg h.s.
Centrally acting agents		
Clonidine		
• Catapress	0.1 mg b.i.d.	1.2 mg b.i.d.
• Catapress TSS patches	0.1 mg/d (applied weekly)	0.6 mg/d (applied weekly)
Methyldopa (Aldomet)	250 mg b.i.d.	1500 mg b.i.d.
Diuretics		
Hydrochlorothiazide "HCTZ" (HydroDiuril, Microzide)	12.5–25 mg q.d.	50 mg q.d.
Indapamide (Lozol)	1.25 mg q.d.	5 mg q.d.
Vasodilators (direct vasodilators)		
Hydralazine	25 mg b.i.d.	150 mg b.i.d.

[a] Give initial dose at bedtime (in case hypotension or orthostatic hypotension occurs with therapy).

[b] Decrease initial dose in patients on diuretic therapy.

[c] Doses higher than the initial dose are usually given b.i.d.

(Adapted from the Sixth Report of the Joint National Committee on Prevention, Detection, Evaluation, and Treatment of High Blood Pressure. *Arch Intern Med* 1997.)

✪ CLINICAL PEARLS ✪

"Pseudohypertension" due to increased arterial rigidity resulting in falsely high blood pressure determination should be suspected in elderly patients with high measured blood pressure who fail to respond to multiple antihypertensive agents therapy and/or those with antihypertensive therapy who develop symptoms that suggest cerebral hypoperfusion but who continue to have elevated measured blood pressure.

WHEN TO CONSIDER AMBULATORY BLOOD PRESSURE MONITORING

Ambulatory blood pressure monitors take readings every 15 to 30 minutes throughout the day. Readings from ambulatory monitoring have been shown to correlate better with target organ damage than clinic measurements. Situations in which ambulatory monitoring should be considered, as recommended by the Ad Hoc Panel of the American Society of Hypertension, include the following:

- Suspected white coat hypertension
- Apparent drug-resistant hypertension
- Hypotensive symptoms while the patient is receiving antihypertensive medications
- Episodic hypertension
- Autonomic dysfunction.

WHEN TO CONSIDER EVALUATING PATIENTS FOR SECONDARY HYPERTENSION

Most patients with hypertension have "primary" or "idiopathic" hypertension and, other than the evaluation described in the preceding section, no further evaluation of their hypertension is necessary. However, a minority of patients with hypertension will have an identifiable cause ("secondary hypertension"). Patients in whom secondary hypertension should be suspected, and for whom additional tests or studies should be considered, include patients:

- Whose initial evaluation suggests secondary causes
- Who respond poorly even to multiple antihypertensive agents
- With previously well-controlled hypertension whose blood pressure abruptly increases
- With stage 3 hypertension
- With sudden onset of hypertension.

Selected symptoms and findings, and the secondary cause of hypertension they suggest, are listed in Table 8.7.

Table 8.7. *Selected symptoms and findings and the secondary causes of hypertension they suggest*

Symptoms and/or findings	Condition
Labile or paroxysmal hypertension with headache, palpitations or perspiration	Pheochromocytoma
Abdominal bruits (especially when lateralized or with diastolic component)	Renal artery stenosis
Abdominal or flank mass	Polycystic kidneys
Decreased blood pressure in lower extremities and decreased and/or delayed femoral pulses	Coarctation of the aorta
Elevated creatinine and/or abnormal urinalysis	Renal parenchymal disease
Truncal obesity with purple striae	Cushing syndrome
Hypokalemia (not due to diuretics)	Primary aldosteronism
Hypercalcemia	Hyperparathyroidism

(Adapted from the Sixth Report of the Joint National Committee on Prevention, Detection, Evaluation, and Treatment of High Blood Pressure. *Arch Intern Med* 1997.)

SUMMARY

Although untreated or inadequately treated hypertension is a major contributor to cardiovascular and renal disease, appropriate treatment can significantly reduce the morbidity associated with this condition. The initial step in the evaluation of the patient who presents with elevated blood pressure is to confirm with several further visits that the patient does have hypertension. Once the diagnosis of hypertension is made, a thorough initial evaluation should be performed with the goals of assessing for target organ damage and cardiovascular disease, identifying other cardiovascular risk factors, and identifying possible secondary causes of hypertension. The patient's stage of hypertension and risk group should be determined in order to guide therapy.

In patients without comorbid conditions that warrant treatment with certain agents, first-line medical therapy should consist of administration of either a diuretic or a beta blocker. In those patients who do not respond to treatment with one agent, the addition of a diuretic (if the patient is not already receiving one) should be strongly considered. Target blood pressure in most patients with hypertension is less than $^{140}/_{90}$ mm Hg. Patients with diabetes mellitus and those with renal parenchymal disease with proteinuria should have blood pressure lowered to less than $^{130}/_{85}$ mm Hg. Patients with established atherosclerosis also should be treated so that their blood pressure is lowered to less than $^{130}/_{85}$ mm Hg, provided they tolerate the lowering of blood pressure to this level. Elderly patients with isolated systolic hypertension benefit from antihypertensive therapy and should receive antihypertensive therapy similar to that given to other patients with hypertension.

9

Treatment Guidelines for Patients with Hypercholesterolemia

Glenn N. Levine

Baylor College of Medicine, Cardiac Catheterization Laboratory, Houston V. A. Medical Center, Houston, Texas 77030

Hypercholesterolemia is a major risk factor for the development of atherosclerosis and clinical ischemic heart disease. The results of several recent studies have now conclusively demonstrated that treatment of hypercholesterolemia, particularly elevated low-density-lipoprotein (LDL) levels, with lipid-lowering medication can decrease the risks of future cardiac ischemic events and can, in fact, significantly decrease overall mortality. In this chapter, the evaluation and management of patients with elevated cholesterol levels, based in part on recommendations issued by the National Institutes of Health's (NIH) expert panel for the National Cholesterol Education Program (NCEP), are discussed.

✪ CLINICAL PEARLS ✪

The total cholesterol level is determined primarily by three lipid levels: LDL cholesterol, high-density lipoprotein (HDL) cholesterol, and triglycerides. It can be calculated from the following formula (as long as the triglyceride level is not greater than 400 mg/dL):

$$Total\ Cholesterol = LDL + HDL + Triglyceride/5.$$

PRIMARY AND SECONDARY PREVENTION

The evaluation and treatment of patients with hypercholesterolemia varies depending on whether the patient does or does not have known atherosclerotic disease. Treatment of hypercholesterolemia in subjects without known coronary artery or vascular disease is denoted as "primary prevention." Treatment in patients with known atherosclerotic disease is denoted as "secondary prevention." In both cases, treatment guidelines are based primarily on LDL cholesterol levels.

✪ CLINICAL PEARLS ✪

In contrast to the clear relationship between LDL cholesterol and cardio-vascular disease, the relationship between elevated triglyceride levels and coronary artery disease is complex and still debated. Therefore, at present, the primary goal of treatment of marked elevations of triglyceride levels should be considered to be a reduction in the risk of pancreatitis. In such patients, possible secondary causes, including alcohol abuse, medications, and diabetes, should be assessed. Agents useful in treating patients with markedly elevated triglyceride levels include gemfibrozil (Lopid) and nicotinic acid.

OBTAINING SERUM CHOLESTEROL SAMPLES

In general, initial assays of patients' total cholesterol and HDL cholesterol levels can be obtained in nonfasting patients. However, when measurements of LDL cholesterol are made that will determine the treatment plan in patients, such measurements should be done in the fasting state.

✪ CLINICAL PEARLS ✪

During the convalescence phase after acute myocardial infarction (or other acute illness), there may be a modest fall in lipid levels. Therefore, in such patients, lipid levels should ideally be obtained within 24 hours of admission or 6 to 12 weeks after hospital discharge. It should be noted, however, that if lipid levels are obtained between these two time periods and are elevated, then the patient should be considered to have hyper-cholesterolemia, and treatment should be initiated.

The NCEP suggests obtaining two measurements of LDL levels 1 to 8 weeks apart. It further suggests that if the two measurements vary by more than 30 mg/dL, a third level be obtained, and the average of all three measurements used. This may prove impractical in some clinical settings, and in clinical practice many practitioners will use only one measurement.

GENERAL CONSIDERATIONS IN PATIENTS WITH HYPERCHOLESTEROLEMIA

Several steps should be undertaken in the evaluation and management of all patients with hypercholesterolemia.

Patient Evaluation

Most cases of hypercholesterolemia have no clear precipitant causes. However, several conditions and medications can lead to elevated lipid levels, and some of these causes can be addressed. Medical conditions associated with hypercholesterolemia include diabetes mellitus, hypothyroidism, nephrotic syndrome, and obstructive liver disease. Drugs that can cause hypercholesterolemia include anabolic steroids, corticosteroids, progestins, and thiazide diuretics.

Dietary Therapy

All patients with hypercholesterolemia should undergo dietary counseling and be started on a low-cholesterol diet. The most important aspect of dietary modification is a reduction of *saturated fat* intake, because it is saturated fats that raise LDL more than any other component of the diet. Adherence to the American Heart Association (AHA) Step II diet may reduce LDL levels by 10% to 20%. Important points to emphasize to the patient regarding changes in diet are summarized in Table 9.1.

Physical Activity

Regular aerobic physical activity may lead to weight loss, a modest decrease in LDL level, and a modest increase in HDL level. All patients should be encouraged to engage in a degree of regular aerobic physical activity appropriate to their overall health status.

Weight Control

Even modest degrees of weight loss in overweight patients can aid in lowering LDL cholesterol. This point should be emphasized to patients, and

TABLE 9.1. *Important points to emphasize to patients regarding changes in diet*

- Emphasize the consumption of fruits, vegetables, breads, cereals, rice, legumes, and pasta
- Minimize consumption of commercially prepared and processed food (cakes, cookies, etc.)
- Eat *lean* fish, poultry, and meat. Remove the skin from chicken and trim the fat from beef before cooking
- Use skim or 1% milk
- Avoid breaded, fried foods
- Eat no more than two egg yolks (or whole eggs) per week
- Use vegetable oils that are high in *unsaturated* fat (corn, olive, canola, and safflower oil)
- Use *soft* margarines (the softer the margarine, the more unsaturated it is)

all overweight patients should be instructed to design a plan for weight loss.

Estrogen replacement therapy in postmenopausal women can lead to lower total and LDL cholesterol levels, and a modest elevation in HDL levels. Because estrogen replacement therapy in general has been associated with lower cardiovascular event rates, it should be particularly considered in postmenopausal patients with hypercholesterolemia.

PRIMARY PREVENTION

The algorithms for the evaluation and treatment of individuals without known atherosclerosis developed by the NCEP actually are quite complex, and a complete discussion of these algorithms is beyond the scope of this book. These algorithms call for multiple measurements of lipid levels at different times, which may prove impractical in some cases. A more simplified algorithm is presented in Fig. 9.1. (Those wishing to obtain the complete algorithms should call 301-251-1222 and request a copy of NIH Publication No. 93-3095, "Second Report of the Expert Panel on Detection, Evaluation, and Treatment of High Blood Cholesterol in Adults," or access the NHLBI web site at www.nhlbi.nih.gov/nhlbi/nhlbi.hpm.)

Screening Recommendations

It is recommended by the expert panel that total cholesterol as well as HDL cholesterol be measured at least once every 5 years in all individuals 20 years of age or older. You may want to measure the LDL level (if the patient is in the fasting state) at the same time because treatment decisions will be based mainly on the LDL level.

Initial Treatment Recommendations

Dietary therapy and lifestyle modification, as outlined in the previous section, should be initiated in those individuals with either:

- LDL 130–159 mg/dL and two or more cardiac risk factors *or*
- LDL ≥160 mg/dL (regardless of the presence or absence of cardiac risk factors).

In general, it is recommended that, for primary prevention, the use of lipid-lowering medications not be considered until the results of a trial of

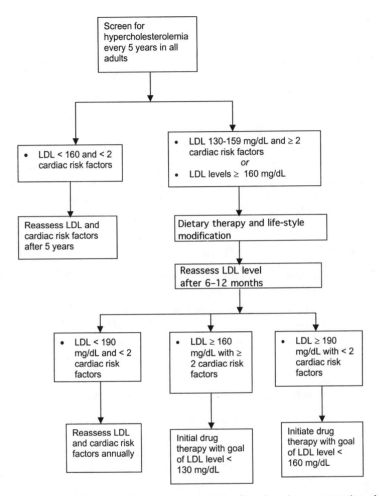

FIG. 9.1. Simplified evaluation and treatment algorithm for primary prevention of atherosclerotic disease.

dietary therapy (and lifestyle modification) are assessed. Levels of LDL should be reassessed after 6 to 12 months of dietary therapy.

When to Consider Medical Therapy

The decision to initiate drug therapy is based on two factors: (i) LDL level (after a trial of dietary therapy) and (ii) presence or absence of two or more cardiac risk factors. Drug therapy should be considered in the following two groups:

- Those with LDL levels ≥160 mg/dL *and* two or more cardiac risk factors
- All those with LDL levels ≥190 mg/dL (regardless of the presence or absence of cardiac risk factors).

There are no definitive guidelines as to which lipid-lowering agent should be prescribed. However, because one recent large trial (the "West of Scotland" study) demonstrated reduced overall mortality with treatment with a 3-hydroxy-3-methylglutaryl coenzyme A (HMG-CoA) reductase inhibitor and because these agents are easy to use and are the most potent LDL lowering drugs available, such agents appear a reasonable first-line therapy.

Treatment Goals

The goals of drug therapy depend primarily on the presence or absence of two or more cardiac risk factors. In those with two or more cardiac risk factors, LDL levels should be reduced to less than 130 mg/dL. In those with less than two cardiac risk factors, LDL levels should be reduced to less than 160 mg/dL. The above recommendations are summarized in Table 9.2.

When to Add a Second Lipid-lowering Agent

If the LDL level cannot be lowered to target levels using maximum doses of one agent, a second agent should be used. In those initially treated with a HMG-CoA reductase inhibitor, either a more potent HMG-Co-A reductase inhibitor (such as atorvastatin [Lipitor]) should be tried, or a second lipid-lowering agent will need to be added. The choice of second-line lipid-lowering agent could include nicotinic acid (niacin, Niacinol, Naicor, Nicolar, Slo-Niacin, etc.), a bile sequestrant agent (cholestyramine), or gemfibrozil.

Table 9.2. *Guidelines for consideration of drug therapy and goals of therapy in the primary prevention of atherosclerotic disease based on LDL levels (after a trial of dietary therapy) and the presence or absence of ≥2 cardiac risk factors*

LDL level and cardiac risk factor status	Goal of therapy
LDL level ≥160 with ≥ cardiac risk factors	LDL <130 mg/dL
LDL level ≥190 with <2 cardiac risk factors	LDL <160 mg/dL

LDL, low-density lipoprotein.

SECONDARY PREVENTION

The evaluation and treatment of patients with known coronary artery disease is summarized in the algorithm shown in Fig. 9.2. and is discussed below.

Screening Recommendations

All patients with established coronary heart disease should undergo fasting lipid analysis, including and particularly LDL level determination.

General Considerations

In general, the goal of treatment in most patients with established atherosclerosis is to lower the LDL level to ≤100 mg/dL. The several steps listed in the section "General Considerations in Patients with Hypercholesterolemia" should be undertaken in all patients with LDL levels ≥100 mg/dL.

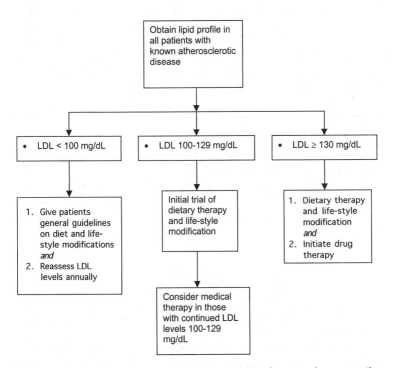

FIG. 9.2. Simplified evaluation and treatment algorithm for secondary prevention of cardiovascular disease.

When to Consider Medical Therapy

Recommendations regarding medical therapy differ depending on whether the patient's LDL level is in the range of 100 to 129 or is ≥130 mg/dL. In patients with LDL levels between 100 and 129 mg/dL, it is recommended that diet and lifestyle modification as described earlier be tried for 6 weeks. In patients who adhere to these recommendations but LDL levels remain between 100 and 129, there are no definitive guidelines as to whether drug therapy should be initiated. Some experts recommend initiating drug therapy with the goal of reducing the LDL level to less than 100 mg/dL in such patients, and the results of a recent large study support this recommendation.

In patients with initial LDL levels ≥130 mg/dL, diet and lifestyle modification alone usually are unlikely to lower LDL levels to less than 100 mg/dL. Therefore, in addition to prescribing dietary and lifestyle modification, drug therapy should be initiated. Although many different classes of lipid-lowering agents are available, the most potent LDL-lowering agents are the HMG-CoA reductase inhibitors ("statins"). It is these agents that have been used in recent trials that have demonstrated reduced morbidity and overall mortality. Therefore, it is reasonable to view these agents as the initial agents of choice in treating patients. As described later, the dose of the HMG-CoA reductase inhibitor that is prescribed should be increased as needed to lower LDL levels to less than 100 mg/dL. Once the appropriate dose is defined, this dose of the medication should be continued indefinitely.

When to Add a Second Lipid-lowering Agent

If the LDL level cannot be lowered to less than 100 mg/dL using the maximal dose of an HMG-CoA reductase inhibitor, either a more potent HMG-CoA reductase inhibitor (such as atorvastatin) should be tried, or a second lipid-lowering agent will need to be added. This second lipid-lowering agent should be either a bile acid sequestrant, nicotinic acid (niacin, Niacinol, Naicor, Nicolar, Slo-Niacin, etc.) or gemfibrozil.

✪ CLINICAL PEARLS ✪

A plethora of educational material is available to patients with hyper-cholesterolemia. One excellent pamphlet, "Live Healthier, Live Longer: Lowering Cholesterol for the Person with Heart Disease," produced by the National Heart, Lung, and Blood Institute (NHLBI) of the NIH can be obtained by patients at no charge by calling the NHLBI Information Center at 301-251-1222 or via their web site at www.nhlbi.nih.gov/nhlbi/nhlbi.hpm.

USING AN HMG-COA REDUCTASE INHIBITOR

Because the HMG-CoA reductase inhibitors (or "statins") appear in general to be the best first-line agents for primary prevention in many patients and for secondary prevention in virtually all patients, the recommended use of these agents will be briefly discussed.

Actions

The statins act primarily by lowering LDL levels. They also lead to modest increases in HDL levels and modest decreases in triglyceride levels.

Prescribing Recommendations

Most of the statins lead to comparable degrees of LDL lowering. The exception to this is the newer agent atorvastatin, which may lower LDL levels to a somewhat greater degree than the other statins. Patients should be started on the lowest initial recommended dose. In general, lipid levels should be reevaluated after 6 weeks of initial therapy. The dose of the prescribed agent should be increased if the LDL level is still ≥100 mg/dL. The LDL level should be reassessed 6 weeks after any dose increases to assess if further dose increases are necessary. The initial and maximum doses of the currently available statins are listed in Table 9.3.

Side Effects

The statins are associated with a low incidence of elevation in serum transaminases (serum glutamic-oxaloacetic transaminase and serum

Table 9.3. *Initial and maximal doses of the currently available HMG-CoA reductase inhibitors ("statins")*

Generic name	Brand name	Initial dose	Maximal dose	Special prescribing considerations
Atorvastatin	Lipitor	10 mg p.o. q.d.	80 mg p.o. q.d.	Can be taken any time of the day
Cerivastatin	Baycol	0.3 mg p.o. q.d.	0.4 mg p.o. q.d.	Should be taken in the evening
Fluvastatin	Lescol	20 mg p.o. q.d.	40 mg p.o. q.d.	Should be taken at bedtime
Lovastatin	Mevacor	20 mg p.o. q.d.	80 mg p.o. q.d.	Should be taken with the evening meal
Pravastatin	Pravachol	10 mg p.o. q.d.	40 mg p.o. q.d.	Should be taken at bedtime
Simvastatin	Zocor	10 mg p.o. q.d.	80 mg p.o. q.d.	Should be taken in the evening

glutamic-pyruvic transaminase). Therefore, liver function tests, particularly transaminase levels, should be assessed before and during therapy. Although suggested regimens vary slightly from statin to statin, a general rule of thumb is to check liver function tests 6 and 12 weeks after initiating therapy, 6 and 12 weeks after dose increases, and periodically (semiannually) thereafter. These liver function tests can be obtained at the same time that lipid levels are being obtained.

The statins also are associated with a very low incidence of myopathy (approximately 1/1,000). It is not necessary to routinely check creatinine phosphokinase levels. However, patients should be instructed to report symptoms of muscle aches or weakness, or if the urine turns brown (which could be a sign of rhabdomyolysis). In patients with such symptoms, the creatinine phosphokinase level should be checked.

⟐ CLINICAL PEARLS ⟐

Concurrent use of nicotinic acid with a statin increases the incidence of liver function test elevation and myopathy. Concurrent use of gemfibrozil with a statin increases the risk of myopathy. Therefore, patients treated with such combination therapy should be monitored closely.

Contraindications to Use

Because the statins may lead to elevated liver transaminase levels, statins should not be prescribed in patients with active liver disease or unexplained elevated transaminases.

SUMMARY

Studies have now definitively demonstrated that treatment of patients with hypercholesterolemia, particularly those with elevated LDL levels, can reduce cardiac morbidity and overall mortality. All adults should be screened for hypercholesterolemia. Treatment decisions for the primary prevention of atherosclerotic disease and are based on LDL levels and the presence or absence of two or more cardiac risk factors. In patients with known atherosclerosis and LDL levels of 100 to 129 mg/dL, dietary therapy and lifestyle modification are suggested. One recent study suggests that medical therapy should also be initiated. In patients with LDL levels ≥130 mg/dL, drug therapy, in addition to diet and lifestyle modification, is indicated, with the goal of lowering LDL levels to less than 100 mg/dL. The HMG-CoA reductase inhibitors should be considered as a first-line agent for primary prevention, and they appear to clearly be the agent of choice for secondary prevention.

10

Anticoagulation in Patients with Cardiovascular Disease

W. Robb MacLellan

University of California, Los Angeles School of Medicine,
Los Angeles, California 90095

An increased risk of thromboembolism is associated with many common cardiac disorders, including atrial fibrillation, coronary artery disease, valvular heart disease, and acute myocardial infarction. This complication is responsible for a significant proportion of the morbidity and mortality associated with these disorders. Over the past 20 to 30 years, results of clinical trials that have tested the impact of anticoagulation on these conditions have revolutionized our approach to the prevention and management of thromboembolic disease. This chapter will focus on outpatient oral anticoagulation therapy in patients with cardiovascular disease. Emphasis will be placed on therapy with warfarin, the mainstay of oral anticoagulant therapy, and provide concise guidelines for the management of most of the commonly encountered clinical situations.

DOSING OF WARFARIN

Although warfarin is rapidly and reliably absorbed, the dose response differs significantly from patient to patient. Its effect on coagulation must be monitored closely until individual dosages are determined. "Loading doses" of warfarin are not necessary and may result in an increased risk of complications. In most patients, an initial daily dose of 5 mg is reasonable. Very frail or elderly patients may be started on lower doses (approximately 2 mg daily).

MONITORING ANTICOAGULATION THERAPY

International Normalized Ratio

Over the last several years, the international normalized ratio (INR) has replaced the prothrombin time as the standard for monitoring oral anticoagulation.

Effects of Warfarin on the International Normalized Ratio

Because the vitamin K-dependent clotting factors affected by warfarin have varying half-lives and clearance, the INR initially becomes elevated in response to the loss of factor VII, which has the shortest half-life of 5 hours. Practically, this means that the INR may overestimate the degree of anticoagulation when therapy is first initiated. However, as the other vitamin K-dependent factors are affected, the INR more accurately reflects the degree of anticoagulation.

Monitoring the International Normalized Ratio

Practical matters dictate that INR monitoring of inpatients and outpatients vary somewhat.

Inpatients

For inpatients, daily INRs should be obtained until the INR remains in the desired therapeutic range for at least 2 consecutive days. Then INRs can be monitored once a week for several weeks and then every 4 to 6 weeks for long-term monitoring.

Outpatients

For outpatients, after initiating therapy, the first INR should be checked approximately 3 days later. Subsequent INRs should be checked weekly until the target range is achieved. Once the target range is achieved, INRs should be checked approximately every 4 to 6 weeks.

Studies have suggested that specialized anticoagulation clinics can improve the safety and effectiveness of anticoagulation therapy while reducing the complications and costs of this therapy when compared with conventionally treated patients. Therefore, uncomplicated patients should be referred to these clinics whenever available.

◯ CLINICAL PEARLS ◯

Recently, the Food and Drug Administration has approved a home anti-coagulation monitoring system based on a simple "finger-stick" device. These will be particularly beneficial in patients who do not have easy access to conventional laboratories and patients whose INRs are unusually difficult to control.

Effects of Drugs and Food on the International Normalized Ratio

Many drugs influence the bioavailability or effects of warfarin, so caution should be exercised whenever initiating new medications in patients already on anticoagulant therapy. A list of medications and food that can affect the INR are given in Table 10.1. You may want to copy this list and give the patient a copy. Whenever any of these medications are started or stopped, more frequent monitoring of the INR for several weeks should be considered.

STOPPING WARFARIN IN PATIENTS UNDERGOING SURGICAL PROCEDURES

There are no definitive guidelines for the management of patients on oral anticoagulation who require elective surgery. Perioperative management must balance the risk of bleeding with risk of thrombosis and systemic

TABLE 10.1. *Selected commonly used medications and selected foods that affect INR*

Medications that can increase INR	Medications and foods that can decrease INR
Amiodarone	Carbamezepine
Omeprazole	Cholestyramine and colestipol
Antibiotics	Phenytoin
• Fluoroquinolones	Rifampin
• Metronadazole	Green leafy vegetables, including
• Trimethoprim-sulfa	• Broccoli
• Certain second- and	• Brussel sprouts
third-generation	• Collards
cephalosporins	• Lettuce
Nonsteroidal anti-	• Spinach
inflammatory agents	• Raw cabbage (cole slaw)
Thyroxine	Herbal products
Herbal products	

emboli. Anticoagulation must be reversed for most types of surgery; however, minimally invasive procedures such as dental cleaning usually can be done with the patient anticoagulated.

Surgery normally can be performed safely once the INR has fallen below 1.5, which occurs approximately 4 days after discontinuation of warfarin in patients whose INR is between 2.0 and 3.0.

For most cardiovascular conditions, it is reasonable to stop the warfarin 3 to 4 days prior to the planned elective surgery. If the patient is already admitted to hospital, preoperative coverage with intravenous heparin can be started when the INR falls below 1.5 (although admission to hospital is not necessary in most cases). The heparin should be discontinued 6 hours prior to surgery. In the absence of overt bleeding it normally is safe to restart the heparin without a bolus 12 hours after the surgery and continue it until reinitiation of warfarin therapy results in an INR above 2.0. In cases where the risk of thromboembolism is low, such as nonvalvular atrial fibrillation and bileaflet aortic mechanical heart valves, postoperative heparin may not be necessary and reinitiation of warfarin therapy may be sufficient.

Elective surgery after venous or arterial thromboembolism should be delayed until at least after the first month because of the high rate of recurrence.

❍ CLINICAL PEARLS ❍

The use of a low molecular weight heparin that can be administered subcutaneously such as enoxaparin (Lovenox) or dalteparin (Fragmin), may prove to be a useful bridge when stopping or restarting anticoagulation therapy with warfarin.

ADVERSE EFFECTS OF WARFARIN THERAPY

Primary care providers should be familiar with several adverse effects of warfarin therapy, the most common of which is bleeding.

Bleeding

Bleeding is the primary complication of anticoagulant therapy and, it is directly related to the intensity and duration of therapy. The risk of bleeding is increased by concomitant treatment with antiplatelet agents, age older than 65 years, history of gastrointestinal bleeding, or serious comorbid medical illness. Added caution should be exercised both in the decision to initiate and in the monitoring of such patients.

Skin Necrosis

Skin necrosis associated with warfarin use is a result of a paradoxical hypercoagulative state associated with widespread thrombosis of small vessels within the subcutaneous fat. It has been associated with rapid oral anticoagulation using high doses of warfarin or protein C or S deficiency. In patients who develop this complication, warfarin therapy should be stopped and heparin therapy initiated.

Embryopathy

Warfarin causes characteristic embryopathy during the first trimester and thus is contraindicated in pregnant patients as well as those who are trying to conceive. Women contemplating pregnancy who require long-term anticoagulation should be switched to heparin prior to trying to conceive.

TREATMENT OF EXCESSIVE ANTICOAGULATION

Treatment of excessive anticoagulation is dependent on the absolute elevation of the INR and the presence or absence of bleeding. In the absence of bleeding, INRs above the normal range but below 5 can be treated conservatively by simply lowering the dose or omitting a dose with reinstitution of anticoagulation therapy at a lower dose. International normalized ratios above 5.0 but below 9.0 can be treated by temporarily holding the warfarin and administering 1 mg of vitamin K orally. International normalized ratios between 9.0 and 20 should be treated with a higher dose of vitamin K (3 to 5 mg) orally. International normalized ratios above 20 should be treated with 10 mg of intravenous vitamin K and consideration given to fresh frozen plasma if there is a significant risk of bleeding. Severe or life-threatening bleeding should be treated aggressively with fresh frozen plasma or prothrombin complex and 10 mg of intravenous vitamin K (which can be repeated if necessary).

NATIVE VALVULAR HEART DISEASE

Rheumatic Mitral Valvular Disease

Rheumatic mitral valvular disease is associated with an increased risk of systemic embolism, even in the absence of atrial fibrillation. The incidence of clinically detectable emboli has been reported to range between 9% and 27% during the course of the disease. This risk is increased with age, left atrial size, or the onset of atrial fibrillation. It is recommended that all patients with rheumatic mitral valvular disease and either history of systemic emboli, left atrial size greater than 5.5 cm, or atrial fibrillation receive full anticoagulation with a target INR of 2.0 to 3.0.

Other Valvular Heart Disease

There is no indication to anticoagulate patients with mitral valve prolapse, aortic valve disease, patent foramen ovale, or atrial septal defects unless associated with systemic emboli or atrial fibrillation.

PROSTHETIC HEART VALVES

The risk of thromboembolic events, and recommendations regarding anticoagulation, depend on the type of prosthetic heart valve and certain clinical factors. Factors that place the patient at higher risk of thromboembolism include:

- Age older than 70 years
- History of previous systemic embolization
- Presence of atrial fibrillation
- Left ventricular dysfunction
- Valve in the mitral position
- Presence of an earlier generation valve (e.g., Starr-Edwards "ball-and-cage" valve)
- Presence of more than one prosthetic valve.

Detailed recommendations for anticoagulation intensity with prosthetic valves are outlined in Table 10.2.

Mechanical Heart Valves

Mechanical heart valves require lifelong anticoagulation because of their high thrombogenic potential. For the currently most commonly implanted mechanical valve, the St. Jude bileaflet tilting-disc valve, the recommended INR is 2.0 to 3.0. In patients with any of the higher-risk characteristics, the INR should be 2.5 to 3.5.

Porcine Bioprosthesis

The risk of thromboembolism with porcine bioprostheses ("pig valves") is mainly limited to the first 3 months; therefore, low-intensity anticoagulation should be instituted during this time (INR 2.0 to 3.0). After this time, no therapy is required unless the patient has a thromboembolic event. Note, however, that some investigators recommend long-term

TABLE 10.2. *Recommendations regarding anticoagulation in patients with prosthetic heart valves*

Valve type	Patients without high risk characteristics (target INR)	Patients with high thromboembolism risk[a] (target INR)
Mechanical valves		
• Newer-generation valves, i.e., St. Jude bileaflet tilting disc	2.0–3.0	2.5–3.5 or 2.0–3.0 + ASA
• Older-generation valves, i.e., Star Edwards "ball and cage"	2.5–3.5	3.0–4.0 or 2.5–3.5 + ASA
Porcine bioprosthetics	2.0–3.0 for 3 months then ASA	2.0–3.0
Homografts	No warfarin	2.0–3.0 for 3 months then ASA

[a] Risk factors include age >70y, history of previous systemic embolization, presence of atrial fibrillation, left ventricular dysfunction, valve in the mitral position, or presence of more than one prosthetic valve.

ASA, acetylsalicylic acid (aspirin).

treatment with aspirin once warfarin is discontinued (although there are no clinical data to support this).

Human Homografts

Human homografts have a very low risk of thromboembolism. Routine anticoagulation, even early postoperatively, is not recommended.

ATRIAL FIBRILLATION

The rationale for antithrombotic therapy with atrial fibrillation (AF) stems from the approximately sixfold increase in risk of stroke compared to people without AF. However, both high-risk and low-risk subgroups exist among patients with AF, which necessitates tailoring therapy to risk. The presence of certain clinical risk factors, shown in Table 10.3, increases the risk of stroke dramatically. Conversely, patients under the age of 65 years without any of these risk factors have a very low annual stroke rate of only 1%.

✪ CLINICAL PEARLS ✪

Some antiarrhythmic agents used in patients with atrial fibrillation, particularly amiodarone, alter the INR in patients on warfarin, so particular care should be exercised when introducing or discontinuing these medications.

TABLE 10.3. *Clinical risk factors associated with an increased risk of stroke in patients with atrial fibrillation*

- Age >75 yr
- Hypertension
- History of stroke or transient ischemic attack
- Congestive heart failure or a left ventricular ejection fraction <40
- Diabetes
- Prosthetic valves
- Rheumatic valvular disease

Lone Atrial Fibrillation

Patients with none of the factors associated with increased risk of stroke are said to have "lone atrial fibrillation." In these patients who are less than 65 years old, aspirin 325 mg p.o. q.d. is considered adequate therapy. In patients between ages 65 and 75 years without risk factors, the risk of stroke is relatively low so an individual decision, balancing the relatively low risk of stroke against the inconvenience and side effects of any therapy, must be determined for each case. However, some consider warfarin the preferred therapy in those without contraindications.

Patients with Risk Factors for Stroke

Patients with atrial fibrillation and risk factors, which are associated with increased risk of stroke, should be anticoagulated with warfarin unless there are strong contraindications. The target INR should be 2.0 to 3.0.

✪ CLINICAL PEARLS ✪

The risk of thrombosis and emboli in patients with atrial fibrillation significantly increases when the INR falls below 2.0, so care should be taken to always maintain the INR above this level.

ACUTE MYOCARDIAL INFARCTION

There is a high incidence of emboli after anterior wall myocardial infarctions, with reported stroke rates of 2% to 6%. The risk of embolization is considered significant enough to warrant anticoagulation therapy with warfarin when a cardiac echocardiogram shows that the anterior wall and/or apex is akinetic (not moving) or dyskinetic (moving paradoxically), and/or when the echocardiogram detects a mural thrombus in the left ventricle. Patients with acute myocardial infarction with such find-

. ings on echocardiogram obtained 1 to several days after the acute event should be anticoagulated with warfarin for 3 to 6 months. The recommended INR is 2.0 to 3.0. Note, however, that routine anticoagulant therapy after this time period, or for a persistently depressed ejection fraction, is not recommended unless there is a concomitant history of systemic emboli, unexplained strokes of transient ischemic attacks, or atrial fibrillation.

SUMMARY

The long-term management of selected cardiac conditions associated with an increased risk of thromboembolism with oral anticoagulants has resulted in significant reductions in mortality and morbidity. Despite this accumulation of data, concerns over the safety of chronic anticoagulation and increased risk of bleeding have often led clinicians to avoid its use. However, careful selection of patients, adherence to modern treatment guidelines, and careful monitoring has been shown to be both safe and extremely effective.

11

Current Recommendations for the Treatment and Prophylaxis of Infective Endocarditis

Douglas L. Mann

Baylor College of Medicine, Section of Cardiology,
Houston V. A. Medical Center, Houston, Texas 77030

Although infective endocarditis (IE) is a relatively infrequent disease in younger individuals, IE increases progressively after 30 years of age, with the rate of cases in those older than 50 years exceeding 15 cases per 100,000. Approximately 10% to 20% of IE cases occur on prosthetic valves (prosthetic valve endocarditis). Intravenous drug abuse entails an even greater risk for IE than that associated with prosthetic valves or rheumatic heart disease. The rate of IE in this group is 2% to 5% per patient-year. Hospitalized patients who are debilitated and who have indwelling intravenous catheters also represent a group of individuals who are susceptible to IE.

In this chapter, the evaluation and treatment of infective endocarditis is discussed. Recommendations regarding which cardiac abnormalities and which procedures require endocarditis prophylaxis are given at the end of the chapter.

EVALUATION OF THE PATIENT WITH SUSPECTED INFECTIVE ENDOCARDITIS

The initial evaluation of patients with suspected endocarditis includes a careful history and physical examination, baseline laboratory tests, electrocardiogram, chest x-ray film, three sets of blood cultures, and a cardiac echocardiogram (Fig. 11.1).

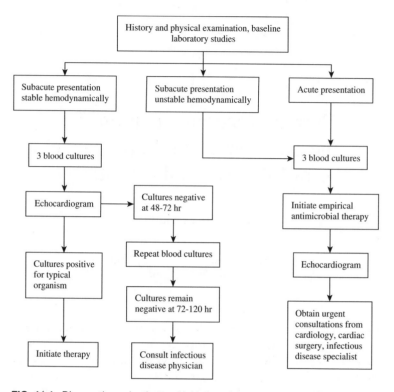

FIG. 11.1. Diagnostic evaluation and initiation of therapy in patients with infective endocarditis. (Adapted from Karchmer AW. Approach to the patient with infective endocarditis. In: Goldman L, Braunwald E, eds. *Primary cardiology*, 1st ed. Philadelphia: WB Saunders, 1998:208.)

Symptoms

Infective endocarditis may present with a wide variety of clinical manifestations, ranging from marked systemic toxicity and rapid progression to an indolent prolonged illness with modest fever and toxicity. The actual clinical symptoms for patients presenting with IE are primarily nonspecific and include fever, chills, sweats, anorexia, weight loss, malaise, cough, headache, and muscle aches. The frequency of specific symptoms in patients with IE is given in Table 11.1.

✪ CLINICAL PEARLS ✪

Although the clinical presentation of *acute* IE may be obvious, the clinical presentation of subacute IE may be very inconspicuous. Patients with *subacute* IE may present with a variety of nonspecific complaints such as weight loss, fatigue, and night sweats. They may have minimal or no fever and a normal white count leukopenia. Because of the nonspecific nature of the symptoms, these patients frequently will have already taken nonsteroidal antiinflammatory agents, salicylates, or even broad-spectrum antibiotics, which makes the diagnosis of IE that much more difficult. For this latter group of patients, the primary care provider must be certain to elicit a careful history of analgesic and antibiotic drug use, as well as have a high index of suspicion to make the diagnosis.

Physical Examination

Most of the physical findings caused by endocarditis (see Table 11.1) are not specific for this diagnosis and should be interpreted in the context of the overall clinical presentation. Fever is present in 80% to 85% of patients; however, the fever is usually low grade, rarely exceeding 39.4°C. Note that fever may be absent in the elderly, in patients with heart failure, and in patients with renal failure or severe disability. Heart murmurs are only present in 80% to 85% of patients with IE; thus, the absence

TABLE 11.1. *Signs and symptoms of infective endocarditis*

Symptoms	Percentage of cases
Fever	80–85
Chills	40–75
Sweats	25
Anorexia	25–55
Weight loss	25–35
Malaise	25–40
Cough	25
Stroke	15–20
Headache	15–40
Myalgia/arthralgia	15–30
Back pain	7–10
Confusion	10–20

Signs	Percentage of cases
Fever	80–90
Heart murmur	80–85
Changing or new murmur	10–40
Systemic emboli	20–40
Splenomegaly	15–50
Clubbing	10–20
Osler's nodes	7–10
Splinter hemorrhage	5–15
Janeway lesions	6–10
Retinal lesions (Roth's spots)	4–10

(Adapted from Karchner AW. Infective endocarditis. In: Braunwald E, ed. *Heart disease,* 5th ed. Philadelphia: WB Saunders, 1997:1084.)

of a murmur does not preclude the diagnosis of IE. The physical examination should include a careful search for other findings that are suggestive (although not diagnostic) of IE, including:

- Splinter hemorrhages
- Osler's nodes (small tender nodules on the finger or toe pads)
- Janeway lesions (small hemorrhages on the palms and soles)
- Splenomegaly.

Electrocardiogram

A baseline electrocardiogram should be obtained in all patients with suspected IE. A change in the length of the PR interval in the electrocardiogram suggests extension of the infectious process (annular abscess formation) into the septum of the heart and heralds a poor prognosis.

Chest Radiography

A baseline chest x-ray film should be obtained in all patients with suspected IE. There are no x-ray findings that are diagnostic of IE. However, the chest x-ray film in intravenous drug addicts with IE commonly reveals nodular infiltrates due to septic pulmonary infarcts caused by emboli from the tricuspid and/or pulmonic valves. The presence of pulmonary edema suggests the development of heart failure and heralds a poor prognosis.

Routine Laboratory Tests

Routine laboratory tests that should be ordered in the evaluation of the patient with endocarditis include serum electrolytes, a complete blood count with differential, liver function tests, platelets, international normalized ratio and partial thromboplastin time, and a urinalysis and culture. The finding of hematuria may suggest emboli to the kidneys.

Blood Cultures

Positive blood cultures remain a vital part of the diagnosis and treatment for IE. More than 95% of all blood cultures obtained in IE patients will be positive. Because one of the pathophysiologic hallmarks of IE is a continuous low-grade bacteremia, it is important to obtain multiple sets of blood cultures over a period of time to differentiate IE from the transient bacteremia that may be associated with indwelling intravenous lines.

Three separate sets of blood cultures should be obtained over 24 hours from separate venipuncture sites to identify the causative organism and to demonstrate that the bacteremia is continuous. The primary care provider should be careful to specify that both anaerobic and aerobic blood cultures should be obtained during the evaluation of the patient.

Organisms that Cause Infective Endocarditis

There are a wide variety of organisms that can cause IE on native and prosthetic heart valves (Table 11.2). Nonetheless, it is worth emphasizing that *Streptococcus viridans* and *Staphylococcus aureus* account for approximately 85% of the infections on native cardiac valves. Thus, a "bacteremia" with a typical organism in an individual with a high likelihood of developing the disease (see following) should always raise the suspicion of IE.

Culture-negative Endocarditis

The term "culture-negative" endocarditis refers to the situation in which the patient has the clinical symptoms of IE but persistently negative blood cultures. The most common cause (50% of cases) of culture-negative

TABLE 11.2. *Etiologic agents for infective endocarditis*

Etiologic organism	Percentage of cases
Native valve endocarditis	
Viridans streptococci	60
Staphylococcus aureus	25
Staphylococcus epidermidis	3
Enterococci	5
Pseudomonas	2
Other gram-negative bacteria	3
Fungi	1
Other infectious agents	1
Early prosthetic valve endocarditis (<60 d after surgery)	
Staphylococcus epidermidis	33
Gram-negative bacteria	19
Staphylococcus aureus	17
Diptheroids	10
Candida albicans	8
Streptococci	7
Other infectious agents	2
Late prosthetic valve endocarditis (>60 d after surgery)	
Streptococci	30
Staphylococcus epidermidis	26
Staphylococcus aureus	12
Gram-negative bacteria	12
Enterococci	6
Diptheroids	4
Candida albicans	3

endocarditis is prior antibiotic therapy; however, the primary care provider should be aware that fastidious organisms that can cause IE (e.g., fungi or Rickettsiae) may be relatively difficult to culture.

✪ CLINICAL PEARLS ✪

Although changing classic murmurs have become a time-honored part of the clinical diagnosis of IE, changing murmurs may not be helpful clinically for several reasons. First, a heart murmur may be absent early in the disease process before valvular damage is sufficient to cause regurgitation. Moreover, lesions on the pulmonary and/or tricuspid valve may produce soft inaudible murmurs because of the relatively low pressures on the right side of the heart. Second, the intensity of murmurs will vary directly with the force of contraction of the heart. Thus, many patients who are febrile with a tachycardia may have a change in the intensity of a benign murmur (particularly systolic murmurs) based on the force of contraction of the heart. Third, patients with indwelling sutures (i.e., patients with prosthetic valves) may have infections along the suture line that do not produce a heart murmur. Thus, the primary care provider should not exclude the presence of IE based on the absence of a changing heart murmur in a patient with suspected IE.

Echocardiogram

In patients with suspected endocarditis, an echocardiogram should be obtained. One primary purpose of obtaining the echocardiogram is to detect "vegetations" on the valve leaflets. Note that because the sensitivity of a standard transthoracic cardiac echocardiogram in detecting vegetations in patients with IE is only 45% to 75%, the lack of findings of a vegetation with this test should not be used to rule out endocarditis. In those patients with suspected endocarditis and negative transthoracic echocardiograms, a transesophageal echocardiogram (TEE), which has a sensitivity of 90% to 94%, should be considered. Even a negative TEE should not be used to rule out endocarditis in a patient in whom there is a high clinical suspicion. In patients with suspected prosthetic valve endocarditis, a TEE should be obtained, as the ability of the standard transthoracic echocardiography to assess prosthetics valves for possible infection is poor. In addition to establishing the diagnosis of endocarditis, echocardiography is useful for following the course of complicated endocarditis. For example, transthoracic echocardiography, although less sensitive, remains useful for assessing chamber dimension and for following the severity of regurgitant lesions in patients with known IE. Echocardiography also may be useful for assessing the presence or absence of known complications of IE, including myocardial abscess formation or flail and/or torn valve leaflets.

◆ CLINICAL PEARLS ◆

Although echocardiography is extremely useful for establishing the diagnosis of IE, this technique is not sufficiently sensitive to exclude IE in a patient in whom the clinical suspicion is high. This is because the overall size of the vegetation may be so small in the early phases of endocarditis that it is below the limits of resolution of the TEE. Alternatively, it may be difficult to clearly discern the presence of vegetations along the sewing rings of prosthetic valves. Among patients in whom there is an intermediate level of suspicion, a negative TEE does not rule out the diagnosis; on the contrary, further evaluation, including another TEE, is required in this situation. Hence, a negative finding on TEE should not dissuade the primary care provider from initiating treatment if clinical suspicion remains high. Alternatively, the primary care provider may want to seek subspecialty consultation in cases where the diagnosis of IE is suspected but cannot be proven.

DIAGNOSIS OF INFECTIVE ENDOCARDITIS

Diagnostic Criteria

A recently described set of major and minor criteria, which incorporates advances in imaging techniques, should now be utilized in making the diagnosis of endocarditis. These criteria are given in Table 11.3. The finding of two major criteria, one major and three minor criteria, or five minor criteria allows a definite diagnosis of IE to be made. Note that occasionally patients may fall just short of the diagnosis of definite IE and yet have no alternative diagnosis to explain their febrile illness. These patients should be classified as possibly having IE and should be treated as if they have IE.

MANAGEMENT OF INFECTIVE ENDOCARDITIS

Objective in Treating Patients

There are two major objectives in treating patients with endocarditis. The first is to eradicate the infecting organism. Failure to accomplish this results in a relapse of the infection. The second is to assess the degree of valve destruction resulting from IE and to institute appropriate therapy when indicated. The diagnosis and management for patients with valvular heart disease is reviewed in Chapter 4. Accordingly, the remainder of this section will focus on antimicrobial therapy for IE.

TABLE 11.3. *Proposed clinical criteria for diagnosis of infective endocarditis*

The diagnosis of definite endocarditis may be made if the following constellation of criteria are present: two major, one major criterion and three minor criteria, or five minor criteria.

A. Major criteria
- Positive blood culture
  - Two separate blood cultures yielding organisms typical for infective endocarditis
  or
  - Microorganisms consistent with infective endocarditis from persistently positive blood cultures
- Evidence for cardiac involvement
  - Positive echocardiogram of infective endocarditis
    - Mobile mass on a native or prosthetic valve
    - New or partial valvular dehiscence of a prosthetic valve
    - Myocardial abscess
  or
  - New valvular regurgitation (worsening or changing of preexisting murmur is not diagnostic)

B. Minor criteria
- Predisposing heart condition (see Table 11.5)
- Fever >38.0°C
- Vascular phenomena: arterial emboli, mycotic aneurysm, intracranial hemorrhage, conjunctival hemorrhages, Janeway lesions
- Immunologic phenomena: glomerulonephritis, Osler's nodes, Roth's spots, rheumatoid factor, elevated erythrocyte sedimentation rate
- Microbiologic: Consistent with infective endocarditis but not meeting a major criterion (one positive culture with typical organism or serologic evidence of an infection with a typical organism)
- Echocardiographic findings: Consistent with infective endocarditis but not meeting a major criterion (see above)

Antibiotic Therapy

Effective antimicrobial therapy requires the use of an agent or combination of agents that is *bactericidal* (not bacteriostatic) for the causative organism. The regimens recommended for therapy are based on the precise susceptibility of the causative organism and prior clinical experience in the treatment of IE caused by the organism. Although a complete description of the principles of antibiotic therapy is beyond the intended scope of this text, the primary care provider should be aware of the sensitivity of the organism to the various antibiotic therapies listed.

The consensus regimens recommended for the treatment of the common bacterial causes of IE are similar for patients with infection of native valves (Table 11. 4). The treatment strategies for more virulent organisms and/or for prosthetic valve endocarditis are beyond the intended scope of this chapter. Such strategies should be developed with consultative support from an infectious disease specialist and a cardiologist.

However, if the patient presents acutely ill, it may not be appropriate to wait a full 24 hours to draw blood cultures before initiating therapy. For

TABLE 11.4. *Antibiotic treatment of commonly encountered organisms in infectious endocarditis*

Organism category	Regimen	Penicillin-allergic
Penicillin-sensitive streptococci (e.g., *S. bovis*)	Penicillin G-2 million units I.V. q6h × 4 wk or 2 million units I.V. q6h × 2 wk plus gentamicin 1 mg/kg (max 80 mg) i.v. q8h × 3 wk	Cefetriaxone 2 g I.V. q24h or vancomycin 15 mg/kg I.V. q12h × 4 wk plus gentamicin 1 mg/kg (max 80 mg) I.V. q8h × at least 2 wk
Penicillin-tolerant streptococci (e.g., *S. mutans*)	Penicillin G 2 million units I.V. q6h × 4 wk plus gentamicin 1 mg/kg (max 80 mg) I.V. q8h × 2 wk	Vancomycin and gentamicin as above
Penicillin-resistant streptococci (e.g., enterococci)	Ampicillin G 4 million units I.V. q6h × 6 wk plus gentamicin 1 mg/kg (max 80 mg) I.V. q8h × 4–6 wk	Vancomycin 15 mg/kg I.V.q12h × 6 wk plus gentamicin 1 mg/kg (max 80 mg) I.V. q8h × 6 wk
Staphylococcus aureus	Nafcillin 2g I.V. q4h × 4–6 wk plus gentamicin 1 mg/kg (max 80 mg) for initial 3–5 d If methicillin resistant; vancomycin 15 mg/kg I.V. q12h × 4–6 wk	Cetriaxone 2 8 I.V. q241t hours × 6 wk plus gentamicin 1 mg/kg (max 80 mg) I.V. q8h × 4–6 wk
Staphylococcus epidermidis	Vancomycin 15 mg/kg I.V. q12h × 6 wk plus rifampin 300 mg q8h × 6 wk plus gentamicin 1 mg/kg (max 80 mg) I.V. q8h initial 2 wk	

these acutely ill patients, blood cultures should be obtained immediately, followed immediately by initiation of antibiotic therapy (see following).

Initiating Therapy

The timing for initiating antimicrobial therapy may be critical, depending on the clinical status of the patient at the time of presentation. Patients who present highly toxic and/or with severe hemodynamic decompensation should have blood cultures drawn at the time of presentation and then empirical broad-spectrum antibiotic therapy initiated immediately thereafter.

In patients who are hemodynamically stable and do not appear to be acutely ill, the initiation of antimicrobial therapy empirically before blood cultures have yielded a causative organism may be counterproductive. It is prudent to delay therapy for several days in these hemodynamically stable patients while waiting for the results of the initial blood cultures. It is unlikely that empirical therapy initiated a few days earlier will prevent complications.

Obtaining Consultative Support

Despite appropriate treatment with potent antibiotics, the mortality rates for various forms of IE range from 10% to 50%. Therefore, consultative support should be enlisted from infectious disease specialists and from cardiologists. In patients with severe valvular infections and/or hemodynamic compromise, consultation with a cardiothoracic surgeon should be obtained. The consultative team will be invaluable in terms of assessing the effectiveness of antibiotic therapy, as well as in the planning of future therapy for the patient with IE, particularly if complications arise.

PREVENTION OF INFECTIVE ENDOCARDITIS

One of the major areas where the primary care provider can make an important impact on IE is in the proper recognition and use of antibiotic prophylaxis to prevent IE in susceptible patients.

Which Lesions Need Antibiotic Prophylaxis

Patients with cardiac abnormalities can be divided into those at low, moderate, and high risk for developing IE (Table 11.5). Antibiotic prophylaxis is not recommended for those at low or negligible risk, but it is recommended for patients at moderate or high risk of developing IE.

TABLE 11.5. *Risk of infective endocarditis associated with common cardiac abnormalities*

Low or negligible risk
- Isolated ostium secundum atrial septal defect
- Prior coronary artery bypass surgery
- Mitral valve prolapse without valvular regurgitation
- Physiologic, functional, or innocent heart murmurs
- Cardiac pacemakers and implanted defibrillators

Moderate risk
- Acquired (degenerative) valvular dysfunction
- Hypertrophic cardiomyopathy
- Mitral valve prolapse with valvular regurgitation or thickened leaflets

High risk
- Prosthetic heart valves
- Prior bacterial endocarditis

❖ CLINICAL PEARLS ❖

One commonly encountered clinical question is the use of antibiotic prophylaxis in the patient with mitral valve prolapse. Although the need for antibiotic prophylaxis in this group of patients remains controversial, the risk for IE in patients with mitral valve prolapse appears to be five to ten times higher than in the general population. Therefore, for patients older than 45 years of age who have evidence of "classic" MVP with thickened leaflets on two-dimensional echocardiography or with clinical evidence of a mitral valve "click" and murmur of mitral regurgitation, antibiotic prophylaxis is warranted. However, patients who have mitral valve prolapse without a thickened valve ("nonclassic" MVP) are considered to be at low risk for the development of IE and, therefore, do not require prophylaxis.

Procedures That Require Prophylaxis

Procedures that are likely to induce bacteremia and thus require antibiotic prophylaxis are listed in Table 11.6. The current regimens recommended for use as prophylaxis for procedures are listed in Table 11.7.

SUMMARY

Infective endocarditis is a potentially life-threatening condition that may present with a wide variety of clinical manifestations. Thus, IE represents both a diagnostic and therapeutic challenge to the primary care provider. The optimal sequence of evaluation and treatment of a patient with suspected IE begins with a careful history and physical examination, followed by laboratory tests, electrocardiogram, chest radiography, blood

TABLE 11.6. *Procedures for which infective endocarditis prophylaxis is suggested*

Respiratory tract
- Surgical operation involving mucosa
- Bronchoscopy with rigid bronchoscope

Gastrointestinal tract
- Endoscopy with biopsy
- Colonoscopy with biopsy
- Sclerotherapy for esophageal varices
- Dilatation of esophageal stricture
- Endoscopic retrograde cholangiography with biliary obstruction
- Biliary tract surgery
- Surgery involving intestinal mucosa

Genitourinary tract
- Prostate surgery
- Cytoscopy
- Urethral dilatation
- Vaginal delivery
- Cervical and/or endometrial biopsy

TABLE 11.7. Regimens for infective endocarditis prophylaxis in adults

Setting	Antibiotic	Regimen[a]
Respiratory tract or esophageal procedures		
• Standard	Amoxicillin	2.0 g p.o. 1 h before procedure
• Unable to take oral medication	Ampicillin	2.0 g i.m./i.v. within 30 min of procedure
• Penicillin-allergic patients	Clindamycin	600 mg p.o. 1 h before procedure or i.v. 30 min before procedure
Genitourinary and gastrointestinal tract procedures		
• Moderate-risk patients	Amoxicillin or ampicillin	Amoxicillin 2.0 g p.o. 1 h before procedure or ampicillin 2.0 g i.m./i.v. 30 min before procedure
• Moderate-risk penicillin-allergic patients	Vancomycin	Vancomycin 1.0 g i.v. infused over 1–2 h and completed within 30 min of procedure
• High-risk patients	Ampicillin + gentamicin	Ampicillin 2.0 g i.v./i.m. + gentamicin 1.5 mg/kg within 30 min of procedure, repeat ampicillin 1.0 g i.v./i.m. or amoxicillin 1.0 g p.o. 6 h later
• High-risk, penicillin-allergic patients	Vancomycin + gentamicin	Ampicillin 2.0 g i.v./i.m. + gentamicin 1.5 mg/kg within 30 min of procedure, repeat ampicillin 1.0 g i.v./i.m. or amoxicillin 1.0 g p.o. 6 h later

[a] For patients in the high-risk group, administer half the dose 6 h after the initial dose.

cultures, and echocardiogram. The timing for initiating antimicrobial therapy depends on the clinical presentation of the patient. For patients who present acutely ill, antibiotic therapy should be initiated immediately after the first set of blood cultures is drawn. For patients with suspected IE who present with an indolent course, it is appropriate to hold antibiotic therapy until three sets of blood cultures have been drawn, organisms identified, and sensitivities obtained. Because of the highly complex and often lethal nature of the clinical course of IE, the primary care physician should always enlist the consultative support of an infectious disease specialist and a cardiologist. Antibiotic prophylaxis for patients at moderate to high risk of developing IE remains a mainstay of therapy following selected upper respiratory tract, genitourinary, and gastrointestinal procedures.

12

Evaluation and Treatment of Patients with Pericarditis, Pericardial Effusions, and Cardiac Tamponade

Douglas L. Mann

Baylor College of Medicine, Section of Cardiology,
Houston V. A. Medical Center, Houston, Texas 77030

Pericarditis, pericardial effusions, and cardiac tamponade may be thought of as a pathophysiologic continuum. Pericarditis or pericardial trauma may produce pericardial effusions, which, although generally clinically silent, may be severe enough to produce cardiac compression with resultant hemodynamic collapse (tamponade). In this chapter we will review the evaluation and management of acute pericarditis, pericardial effusions, and cardiac tamponade.

DIAGNOSIS OF ACUTE PERICARDITIS

Acute pericarditis is a syndrome due to inflammation of the pericardium characterized by chest pain, a pericardial friction rub, fever, and serial electrocardiographic changes.

Symptoms

The chest pain of pericarditis can manifest itself in three different ways: it can mimic the pain of an acute myocardial infarction; it can occur as a sharp pain with deep inspiration; and it can occur synchronously with each heartbeat. Generally the pain is exacerbated by lying supine, coughing, or swallowing, and it is relieved by sitting up or leaning forward.

Electrocardiographic Findings

Changes in the electrocardiogram (ECG) are extremely helpful in diagnosing acute pericarditis and are summarized in Table 12.1. Briefly, there are four stages. In Stage I there is PR-segment depression and ST-segment elevation, which unlike the ST-changes seen with acute myocardial infarction, is concave upward. Stage II occurs several days later and is marked by the return of the ST segments to baseline and T-wave flattening. Stage III is characterized by "flipping" of the T waves that is not associated with loss of R-wave voltage on the ECG. Stage IV is characterized by the return of the T-wave changes to normal. One of the hallmarks of these changes in the ECG is that they occur in multiple leads, as opposed to being confined to the anterior, inferior, or lateral ECG leads.

Physical Examination

The pericardial friction rub is the most important sign of pericarditis, and the diagnosis can be made on this finding alone. The classic pericardial friction rub is described as having three components that are related to

---

❂ CLINICAL PEARLS ❂

Echocardiograms are ordered frequently to look for pericardial effusions in the setting of suspected acute pericarditis. However, although the echocardiogram is useful in diagnosing the size and location of pericardial effusions, it is not a reliable test for diagnosing pericarditis because patients may have pericarditis without a pericardial effusion, and pericardial effusions may occur in the absence of pericarditis. Thus, echocardiography is not necessarily a useful first-line test to diagnose pericarditis.

TABLE 12.1. *Sequence of electrocardiographic changes in pericarditis*

	ECG changes	Time course
Stage I	ST elevation (concave up) usually present in all leads except a VR and V_1, PR-segment depression	Accompanies the onset of pain and lasts from 2 h to 3 wk
Stage II	ST segment returns to normal	Several days after the onset of pain and lasts several weeks
Stage III	Inversion of the T waves	Generally begins by the second or third week and lasts up to several months
Stage IV	Reversion of the T waves to normal	May last up to 3 mo

cardiac motion during atrial contraction, ventricular contraction, and rapid ventricular filling. A three-component rub is heard in approximately 50% of the cases. Sometimes the murmur is less characteristic and has only two components, which gives the murmur its "to-and-fro" quality and may make it difficult to differentiate from the combined murmur of aortic stenosis and insufficiency. The single-component rub is the least common rub heard and may occur in patients in atrial fibrillation. An important feature of the rub is that it frequently comes and goes during different parts of the day. Detection of the rub is aided by applying the stethoscope firmly to the lower edge of the sternum during full expiration with the patient leaning forward.

MANAGEMENT OF ACUTE PERICARDITIS

Determining the Cause

The appropriate management of acute pericarditis begins by searching for the cause of the pericardial irritation and determining whether that underlying disorder requires specific treatment. Thus, the first step in managing pericarditis is to try to treat the underlying cause, if one can be determined. Several of the more important causes of pericarditis are listed in Table 12.2 and include nonspecific (idiopathic) causes, viral infections, neoplastic disease, acute myocardial infarction, uremia, radiation, infection, and certain drugs.

Supportive Therapy

Nonspecific supportive therapy for pericarditis includes bed rest until the pain and fever have subsided. Initial observation (24 to 48 hours) in the hospital is warranted for some patients with acute onset of pericarditis to exclude an associated myocardial infarction or bacterial process and to watch for the development of tamponade, which can occur in as many as 15% of the cases of acute pericarditis.

TABLE 12.2. *Causes of pericarditis*

- Idiopathic (nonspecific)
- Viral infections
- Neoplastic disease
- Acute myocardial infarction
- Uremia
- Radiation
- Drugs (hydralazine, procainamide, phenytoin, isoniazid, penicillin)
- Autoimmune and/or collagen vascular disease (lupus, rheumatoid arthritis)
- Infections (tuberculosis, acute bacterial infection, fungal infection)

Medical Therapy

Symptomatic therapy for pericarditis includes nonsteroidal antiinflammatory agents such as aspirin (650 mg p.o. q4h) or indomethacin (25 to 50 mg p.o. t.i.d.). When the pain is severe and/or does not subside quickly, then a trial of oral steroids is warranted (prednisone 60 to 80 mg p.o. q.d.). If the patient's symptoms subside, then the antiinflammatory agents should be tapered slowly over 5 to 7 days. Antibiotics should be reserved for those cases that are documented to be due to a bacterial infection.

❖ CLINICAL PEARLS ❖

Oral anticoagulants should be discontinued during an episode of acute pericarditis because of the concern of developing hemorrhagic pericardial tamponade. If the patient requires anticoagulation (e.g., because of a mechanical prosthetic valve), then it is safer to maintain the patient on intravenous heparin, which can be reversed quickly with protamine. The patient should be monitored closely and frequent echocardiograms should be obtained to be certain that the effusion is not worsening.

Most cases of pericarditis subside; however, pericarditis may recur in up to 20% to 30% of the patients who respond initially. The majority of these patients can be managed with nonsteroidal or steroid antiinflammatory agents. For those patients who do not respond, colchicine has been tried at starting doses of up to 1 mg p.o. daily with some success.

A simplified algorithm for evaluating and treating patients with pericarditis is shown in Fig. 12.1.

PERICARDIAL EFFUSION

Pericardial effusion may develop as a response to pericardial trauma (e.g., an automobile accident) of the parietal pericardium or from inflammation of the pericardium, as discussed earlier. Pericardial effusions ordinarily do not produce symptoms; however, if the accumulation of fluid is substantial and causes intrapericardial pressure to increase, cardiac compression with resultant cardiac tamponade may develop (see following).

DIAGNOSIS OF PERICARDIAL EFFUSIONS

A small pericardial effusion in the absence of an increase in intrapericardial pericardial pressure may result in no specific physical findings, whereas a large effusion may produce quiet heart sounds or crackles over the lungs fields due to compression of lung parenchyma. Abnormalities

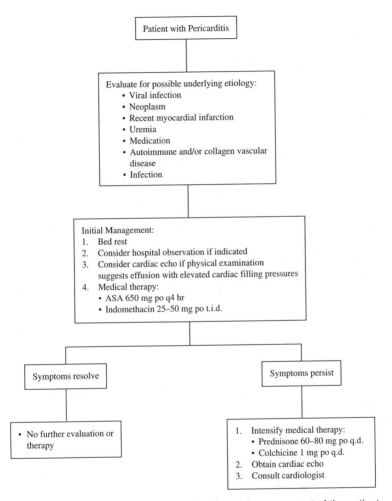

FIG. 12.1. Suggested algorithm for evaluation and management of the patient with pericarditis.

of the arterial pulse, systemic blood pressure, and jugular venous pulse generally do not occur when a pericardial effusion is present without significant elevation of the intrapericardial pressures. The chest x-ray film may not show any enlargement with small pericardial effusions, or an enlarged cardiac silhouette if the effusion is moderate to large in size. The electrocardiographic findings are nonspecific and may include a reduction in the QRS voltage (i.e., less than 5 mm in the limb leads and less than 10 mm in the precordial leads) and/or flattening of the T waves. Rarely, if the effusion is large the height of the QRS complex may alternate with every other beat ("electrical alternans"); however, this finding is rarely seen in current medical practice. Two-dimensional echocardiography is the most useful technique currently available for evaluating pericardial effusions. The accumulation of fluid in the pericardial space results in the appearance of an "echo-free space" around the heart. Depending on the size of the echo-free space around the heart, clinicians will semi-quantitatively assess pericardial effusions as small, moderate, or large.

✿ CLINICAL PEARLS ✿

The rate of accumulation of fluid in the pericardial space, and not necessarily the size of the effusion, will determine whether increased pressures develop in the pericardium. Thus, small effusions that occur rapidly (e.g., after an automobile accident) may be more life threatening than a large effusion that occurs slowly (e.g., in a patient with collagen vascular disease). The primary care provider should not rule out the possibility of a hemodynamically significant effusion based on the size of the effusion alone.

MANAGEMENT OF PERICARDIAL EFFUSIONS

The decision to treat a pericardial effusion is determined by two factors: (i) the nature of the underlying etiology of the pericardial effusion and (ii) whether the effusion causes hemodynamic problems (see section on tamponade following). For example, if the cause of the pericardial effusion is secondary to pericarditis, then the treatment of the effusion is the same as the treatment of the underlying pericarditis. However, if the etiology of the pericardial effusion is unknown and/or the effusion is not causing hemodynamic problems, then there is no compelling reason to treat the pericardial effusion with either antiinflammatory agents or by mechanically removing fluid from the pericardial sac. It bears emphasis that mechanical removal of fluid is not indicated unless there is evidence of pericardial tamponade, or unless an analysis of pericardial fluid is necessary to establish a diagnosis (e.g., malignancy). For many patients with pericardial effusions, the primary care provider can safely assume a "watch and wait policy" rather than embarking on potentially dangerous forms of therapy.

DIAGNOSIS OF CARDIAC TAMPONADE

The most feared consequence of a pericardial effusion is the development of cardiac tamponade, which may lead to life-threatening hypotension as the pressure in the pericardial sac becomes excessively elevated and thereby prevents the heart from filling appropriately. The most frequent causes of cardiac tamponade are neoplasm, idiopathic or viral myocarditis, and uremia, but will vary somewhat depending on the types of patients that the primary care provider sees in clinical practice.

Symptoms

The clinical presentation of patients with cardiac tamponade depends on the rapidity with which the effusion accumulates. For most patients, the pericardial effusion accumulates over a period of weeks to months. When cardiac filling is reduced significantly by the enlarging effusion, patients will appear ill, but not in extremis. The predominant symptom at this point in time may simply be dyspnea. Pleuritic type chest pain may or may not be present, depending on the cause of the effusion.

Physical Examination

Physical examination discloses elevated neck veins, tachypnea, tachycardia, and an inspiratory disappearance of the brachial or femoral pulse (so-called "pulsus paradoxus"). The magnitude of the pulsus paradoxus

---

❖ CLINICAL PEARLS ❖

It is important to recognize that hypotension is a late-presenting feature of cardiac tamponade, especially when the effusion accumulates slowly. Thus, cardiac tamponade can occur with a completely normal blood pressure. There are documented cases of pericardial tamponade where patients have actually been hypertensive at the time that the diagnosis was made! Most patients with cardiac tamponade in whom effusions accumulate slowly will present with nonspecific findings, such as tachypnea and tachycardia. Thus, the primary care provider should not wait until the patient becomes hypotensive to make the diagnosis of cardiac tamponade.

---

can be estimated using the blood pressure cuff. The blood pressure cuff should be inflated 20 mm Hg above the systolic blood pressure and deflated slowly until the first heart sound (Korotkoff sound) is only heard during expiration. The cuff then should be deflated until the Korotkoff sound is heard equally well during inspiration and expiration. The difference between these two pressures is referred to as the pulsus paradoxus. In patients with normal cardiovascular function, a pulsus paradoxus of up to 10 mm Hg is considered normal. Therefore, a pulsus paradoxus greater than 10 mm Hg is considered abnormal by most clinicians. However, it should be recognized that a pulsus paradoxus greater than 10 mm Hg is not specific for cardiac tamponade. It may be seen in patients with asthma, chronic obstructive lung disease, or a large pulmonary embolus. It also should be remembered that a pulsus paradoxus may not be present (i.e., a false-negative) in patients with cardiac tamponade if the patient has concomitant left ventricular hypertrophy, aortic insufficiency, or an atrial septal defect.

✪ CLINICAL PEARLS ✪

In some patients, the pericardial effusion may accumulate over a period of minutes to hours (e.g., after chest trauma from an automobile accident), in which case the clinical presentation generally is quite different from that seen with slowly accumulating effusions. That is, these patients generally will present in extremis, with a low blood pressure and elevated neck veins.

Chest Radiography

There are no x-ray features that are diagnostic of cardiac tamponade. For example, if the effusion accumulates quickly, the cardiac silhouette will appear completely normal, whereas if the effusion accumulates slowly the cardiac silhouette will be enlarged.

Electrocardiographic Findings

The electrocardiographic changes in cardiac tamponade are similar to those discussed earlier for pericarditis and pericardial effusion. Occasionally, with very large pericardial effusions, the height of the ECG will vary from beat to beat (electrical alternans); however, this electrocardiographic finding is encountered infrequently now that effusions are readily diagnosed by two-dimensional echocardiography.

Echocardiographic Findings

As with the diagnosis of pericardial effusions, two-dimensional echocardiography is an extremely useful technique for evaluating cardiac tamponade and should always be ordered, unless the patient is moribund and requires immediate therapy. There are several important findings on two-dimensional echocardiography that are extremely useful in helping to make the diagnosis of cardiac tamponade (Table 12.3). Moreover, the two-dimensional echocardiogram provides critically important information about the location of the effusion, which is important for clinicians

TABLE 12.3. *Echocardiographic findings suggestive of cardiac tamponade*

Right and/or left atrial diastolic collapse
Right ventricular diastolic collapse
Abnormal inspiratory increase in tricuspid valve flow and a >15% inspiratory
decrease in mitral valve blood flow

who will attempt to mechanically remove the fluid from the pericardial space. Nonetheless, it is important to emphasize that none of the echocardiographic findings listed in Table 12.3 are 100% sensitive or 100% specific for cardiac tamponade.

✪ CLINICAL PEARLS ✪

Despite the multitude of diagnostic tests that are available, in most patients the diagnosis of cardiac tamponade remains a clinical diagnosis based on a clinical examination that discloses elevated neck veins, a pulsus paradoxus greater than 10 mm Hg, tachypnea, and tachycardia. The echocardiogram is useful in terms of demonstrating the presence or absence of an effusion and providing useful (although not infallibly diagnostic) information about the hemodynamic significance of the effusion. Right heart catheterization provides confirmatory evidence for "cardiac compression."

Swan-Ganz Catheterization

In this regard it is important to note that right heart catheterization (i.e., Swan-Ganz catheterization) provides extremely useful confirmatory information about the hemodynamic significance of the pericardial effusion and therefore should be considered in all patients in whom the diagnosis of pericardial tamponade is being considered. The diagnostic findings of cardiac tamponade on right heart catheterization are increased diastolic pressures in the heart, with "equilibration" of the diastolic filling pressures in the right atrium, right ventricle, and mean pulmonary capillary wedge pressure (i.e., all the diastolic pressures are equal in all chambers). At the time of this writing there are no firm guidelines that mandate obtaining a right heart catheterization in *all* patients with suspected cardiac tamponade. Thus, the decision to perform a right heart catheterization will be tempered by the hemodynamic status of the patient at the time of evaluation (for example, there may be insufficient time to perform a right heart catheterization if the patient is hypotensive), the degree of certainty with which the clinical and noninvasive diagnosis of tamponade can be made, and the personal preferences of the physician(s) who will mechanically remove fluid from the pericardial sac.

MANAGEMENT OF CARDIAC TAMPONADE

The only treatment that is effective for patients with proven cardiac tamponade is to relieve (i.e., decompress) the cardiac tamponade by removing pericardial fluid. This can be accomplished by (i) percutaneous pericardiocentesis or percutaneous balloon pericardiotomy; (ii) pericardiotomy via a subxiphoid incision; or (iii) surgical removal of the pericardium. A complete discussion of the merits and technical aspects of each of these procedures is beyond the intended scope of this chapter. However, from the perspective of the primary care provider, it cannot be emphasized enough that relieving the cardiac compression through removal of pericardial fluid is the *only* effective long-term means of treating cardiac tamponade. For most primary care providers this will entail *immediately* admitting the patient to a hospital in an intensive care unit setting and *immediately* referring the patient to a cardiologist or surgeon, who will relieve the cardiac compression through one of the procedures outlined earlier. However, until definitive therapy can be performed, the primary care provider can provide important hemodynamic support for the patient by administering intravenous saline, which has been shown to delay (but not prevent) hemodynamic collapse in cardiac tamponade. The use of beta-adrenergic blocking agents should be avoided, because adrenergic drive helps to sustain cardiac output in the setting of cardiac tamponade.

SUMMARY

Pericarditis, pericardial effusions, and cardiac tamponade may be thought of as a pathophysiologic continuum. Most cases of pericarditis are self-limited and respond to nonsteroidal antiinflammatory agents. Pericardial effusions generally are clinically silent and require no specific therapy. However, if the pericardial effusion accumulates sufficiently, then the elevated pressures in the pericardial sac will prevent the heart from filling. If this latter event occurs, hemodynamic collapse will soon follow. Therefore, pericardial effusions that impede filling of the heart, as manifested by elevated neck veins and a pulsus paradoxus, should be treated by mechanically removing fluid from the pericardial space. Whereas the ECG is the most useful diagnostic test in pericarditis, the two-dimensional echocardiogram is the most useful diagnostic test for evaluating pericardial effusions.

13

Management of the Pregnant Patient with Cardiovascular Disease

Sheilah Bernard

*Boston University School of Medicine, Section of Cardiology,
Boston Medical Center, Boston, Massachusetts 02118*

Cardiovascular changes that occur during normal pregnancy can exacerbate preexisting cardiac conditions and thus can be potentially harmful to the mother and/or fetus. An understanding of these changes and of the management of pregnant patients with cardiovascular disease can decrease the chances of adverse outcome during pregnancy. In this chapter, the physiologic changes that occur during pregnancy and with delivery, and the management of patients with specific cardiovascular conditions are discussed.

PHYSIOLOGIC CHANGES DURING PREGNANCY AND DELIVERY

Changes in Blood Components

Total plasma volume increases by approximately 50% and red blood cell volume increases 25% during the 40 weeks of pregnancy. This results in an overall increase in blood volume of 40%. The disproportionate increase in plasma volume accounts for the *physiologic anemia of pregnancy*.

Cardiac Output

Cardiac output increases initially by an increase in stroke volume. Toward the end of pregnancy, the stroke volume normalizes due to decreased blood return resulting from inferior vena caval compression by the gravid uterus. Cardiac output then is maintained by an increase in heart rate.

Vascular Resistance

Systemic vascular resistance falls during pregnancy due to hormonal changes and the creation of a low-resistance circulation in the uterus and placenta.

Delivery

During delivery, uterine contractions cause transient autotransfusions of up to 500 mL of blood into the central circulation, resulting in increased stroke volume and cardiac output. Maternal pain and anxiety during delivery increase sympathetic tone, augmenting the increase in stroke volume and cardiac output. Adequate local or epidural anesthesia should be provided to prevent these sympathetic-mediated stresses on the cardiovascular system. Cesarean section causes less prominent changes in cardiac output, but hemodynamic changes due to anesthesia, blood loss, and relief of caval compression can still occur.

Postpartum

Immediately after delivery, the cardiac output initially is elevated due to release of inferior vena caval compression, but it quickly normalizes. All hemodynamic changes return to normal over the next few weeks.

CARDIOVASCULAR SYMPTOMS AND SIGNS ASSOCIATED WITH PREGNANCY

The physiologic changes that occur during pregnancy can lead to cardiovascular symptoms and abnormal physical findings in otherwise normal patients. Unfortunately, these resultant symptoms and findings can make distinguishing normal physiologic changes from pathologic ones challenging.

Symptoms Associated with Pregnancy

During pregnancy, dyspnea is common due to elevation of the diaphragm and gestational hormonal changes. Lightheadedness and presyncope are caused by decreased vena caval return to the heart. Palpitations are noted frequently as the heart rate increases during pregnancy.

✿ CLINICAL PEARLS ✿

The *supine hypotensive syndrome of pregnancy* is hypotension and bradycardia due to reduced venous return when the patient lies on her back and the fetus and uterus cause inferior vena caval compression. This can be relieved by instructing the patient to lie in the left lateral decubitus position, which displaces the uterus leftward of the inferior vena cava.

Physical Findings Associated with Pregnancy

The physical examination in normal pregnancy can include a laterally displaced PMI due to elevation and rotation of the heart by the gravid uterus. Fluid retention, seen early in the form of elevated neck veins and later as peripheral edema, is a reflection of the increased plasma volume and vena caval compression, respectively. There can be a physiologic S3 due to rapid ventricular filling in the volume-overloaded state. An S4 is an infrequent finding.

Systolic flow murmurs in the aortic and pulmonic areas are commonly grade I–II/VI in intensity due to increased stroke volume across anatomically normal valves. Systolic regurgitant murmurs (mitral and/or tricuspid regurgitation) generally become softer during pregnancy due to decreased systemic vascular resistance. Systolic murmurs louder than grade II/VI, especially radiating to the neck, warrant further studies. Diastolic murmurs, although occasionally representing increased filling volumes across the mitral and tricuspid valves, generally are pathologic and should be investigated.

◆ CLINICAL PEARLS ◆

Two murmurs associated exclusively with pregnancy are the cervical venous hum, a continuous murmur heard best in the right supraclavicular fossa, which can be eliminated by turning the head to the opposite side, and the "mammary souffle," a continuous murmur heard over the breast in late gestation or early postpartum, which can be eliminated by light pressure of the stethoscope.

DIAGNOSTIC CARDIAC TESTING IN PREGNANCY

Electrocardiographic Changes

Electrocardiographic changes during pregnancy include sinus tachycardia, slight axis shifts, and occasional atrial premature beats and/or ventricular premature beats. ST-T wave abnormalities are not routinely seen in pregnancy and should be considered abnormal.

Echocardiographic Testing and Findings

Echocardiograms (two-dimensional and Doppler studies) can be performed safely in pregnancy. Frequent normal findings include chamber dilation due to increased stroke volumes, small pericardial effusions, and mild mitral and tricuspid regurgitation. The findings of moderate or severe mitral and/or tricuspid regurgitation are not normal findings and warrant further investigation

Exercise Stress Testing

Low-level stress testing can diagnose ischemic heart disease and assess maternal functional capacity. Maximal level stress testing is not recommended due to the occurrence of fetal bradycardia at peak maternal heart rates.

Radiographic Procedures

Radiographic procedures are routinely discouraged during pregnancy due to the potential of fetal harm. When chest radiography is necessary, pelvic shielding should be used. Chest x-ray films may demonstrate cardiomegaly and pulmonary vascular congestion due to volume overload. Small pleural and pericardial effusions may be seen. Fluoroscopy also is discouraged, but it can be performed with appropriate shielding of the fetus. Computerized tomography and radionuclide studies should be avoided in the absence of clear data to support their safety. Magnetic resonance imaging is discouraged during the first trimester, but it has not been associated with fetal hazard when used in the evaluation of congenital heart disease and aortic dissection.

PREGNANCY AND PREEXISTING HEART DISEASE: CONGENITAL HEART DISEASE

Patients with congenital heart disease should receive early counseling on maternal/fetal risks to pregnancy, contraceptive alternatives, risk of passing congenital traits to offspring, endocarditis prophylaxis, and/or anticoagulation risks. Consideration should be given to elective repair of lesions prior to pregnancy. In general, patients with acyanotic congenital conditions tolerate pregnancy well. However, patients with arrhythmias, elevated pulmonary vascular resistance, or congestive heart failure should be watched carefully during pregnancy for worsening symptoms.

Left-to-right Shunts

Left-to-right shunts (atrial septal defects and ventricular septal defects) are the most common forms of acyanotic congenital heart disease. Shunting during pregnancy tends to decrease due to the reduction in systemic vascular resistance that occurs during pregnancy.

Eisenmenger's Syndrome

Eisenmenger's syndrome is right-to-left intracardiac shunting due to an elevated and fixed pulmonary vascular resistance. This cyanotic physiology is associated with a high maternal mortality, and pregnancy is contraindicated. Patients should be advised to undergo sterilization; therapeutic abortion should be strongly considered in the pregnant patient with Eisenmenger's syndrome.

Tetralogy of Fallot

Tetralogy of Fallot (right ventricular hypertrophy, overriding aorta, ventricular septal defect, and right ventricular outflow obstruction) is the most common form of cyanotic congenital heart disease surviving to adulthood. Pregnancy is tolerated following surgical correction of the underlying lesion, but residual right ventricular outflow gradients may worsen with symptomatic deterioration.

Aortic Coarctation

Aortic coarctation frequently is corrected prior to child-bearing years. The pregnant patient with corrected aortic coarctation remains at risk for aortic dissection/rupture due to the influence of gestational hormones. The focus of therapy in these patients should be adequate blood pressure control and limitation of physical activity. Surgical repair of the coarctation can be performed emergently for heart failure or severe, uncontrolled hypertension, but medical therapy is preferred if possible. Most aortic dissections occur prior to labor. Patients with coarctations can tolerate vaginal deliveries with good anesthesia.

Hypertrophic Cardiomyopathy

Pregnant women with hypertrophic cardiomyopathy generally become very dyspneic during pregnancy because of the additional volume imposed on the noncompliant ventricle. Symptomatic patients should be managed with judicious diuretics, salt/water restriction, bed rest, and beta blockers to prolong diastole and reduce any provokable left ventricular outflow gradient. Patients who develop atrial fibrillation or other tachyarrhythmias usually tolerate these arrhythmias extremely poorly. Therefore, supraventricular arrhythmias should be rapidly treated by controlling the ventricular response with the use of beta blockers and by promptly reverting the rhythm to sinus rhythm through either antiarrhythmic agents or synchronized cardioversion. Digoxin should not be used for ventricular

TABLE 13.1. Selected cardiovascular medications and the FDA pregnancy categorization

Medication	FDA pregnancy category	Fetal effects	Comments
Angiotensin-converting enzyme inhibitors	D	Neonatal renal failure, low birth weight, premature delivery, oligohydramnios	Contraindicated during pregnancy
Adenosine	C	No change in fetal heart rate or uterine contraction in case reports	No animal or fetal studies have been conducted on possible fetal effects
Amiodarone	D	Congenital hypothyroidism, premature birth, growth retardation, bradycardia	Strongly consider preferentially using other antiarrhythmic agents; not recommended in nursing mothers
Beta blockers Metoprolol/pindolol	B	Intrauterine growth retardation,	Variable transfer to placenta and breast milk
Atenolol/labetalol/ propranolol/nadolol	C	fetal bradycardia, fetal hypoglycemia	
Calcium channel blockers	C	Heart block, hypotension	Associated with higher rate of cesarean sections, premature delivery, and small-for-date infants
Digoxin	C	Low birth weights	Associated with earlier and shorter labor; considered safe in nursing mothers
Disopyramide	C	Low birth weights	Compatible with nursing; may induce uterine contraction/delivery

Drug	Category		
Diuretics			Transfer to placenta; exacerbate preeclampsia by reducing plasma volume;
• Furosemide	C		
• Thiazides	D	Hypoglycemia, hemolytic anemia, thrombocytopenia, hyponatremia, bradycardia	thiazides may inhibit lactation
Heparin	C	None, does not cross placenta	Heparin-induced thrombocytopenia; bleeding and thrombotic complications in mother
Hydralazine	B	Considered safe	Compatible with nursing
Lidocaine	B	Safe when fetal acid-base status is normal	Compatible with nursing
Methyldopa	A	None	Negligible risks
Procainamide	C	No teratogenic reports	Compatible with nursing; maternal lupus-like syndrome with chronic therapy
Quinidine	C	Rare	Compatible with nursing
Warfarin (Coumadin)	D	Coumarin embryopathy (nasal bone hypoplasia, chondrodysplasia punctata) during first 8–12 wk of gestation; fetal bleeding, spontaneous abortion, low birth weight	Contraindicated during first trimester and at term; avoid throughout pregnancy provided alternate anticoagulant therapy achieves adequate maternal protection

rate control, because its inotropic properties could worsen the dynamic outflow tract gradient.

Hypovolemia (such as from excessive diuretic use) should be avoided. Spinal/epidural anesthetics during delivery should be avoided because of their associated vasodilation and subsequent worsening of the outflow tract gradient. Patients with left ventricular outflow tract murmurs should receive endocarditis prophylaxis (Table 13.1).

Marfan's Syndrome

Marfan's syndrome is an autosomal dominant connective tissue disorder characterized by aortic dilation, mitral valve prolapse, and ectopia lentis in a nonhypertensive young person. It is associated with aortic insufficiency due to root dilation and mitral regurgitation due to myxomatous mitral valve. Patients are predisposed to aortic dissection. Preconception counseling should include maternal and fetal risk assessment. Patients are at higher maternal risk if the aorta is dilated prior to pregnancy, and these patients should be advised against pregnancy. Medical measures during pregnancy should include the use of beta blockers and avoidance of physical activity. Elective cesarean section is the preferred route of delivery. Complications of acute aortic dilation or dissection sometimes can be surgically repaired emergently, but at increased fetal risk.

PREGNANCY AND ACQUIRED CARDIAC CONDITIONS

Systemic Hypertension

Ten percent of pregnancies are complicated by hypertension. The diagnosis may be difficult to establish in those who have not sought medical attention before the pregnancy. Any elevated pressure (>140/>90) during the first trimester should be considered essential hypertension and unrelated to the pregnancy itself. In the absence of end-organ damage (retinopathy, nephropathy, left ventricular hypertrophy noted on electrocardiogram), there are no increased risks.

The development of high blood pressure after 20 weeks of gestation is considered gestational hypertension. In patients who already have hypertension, further elevations of blood pressure that occur beyond the 20-week point also should be considered a form of gestational hypertension. Note that maternal and fetal risks increase as the diastolic pressure exceeds 110 mm Hg. Preeclampsia is the syndrome of hypertension, proteinuria, and edema, with or without associated coagulopathy and liver abnormalities, which occurs after 20 weeks.

Treatment of chronic hypertension includes continuation of previously prescribed diuretics, beta blockers, or calcium antagonists. When treatment is initiated or intensified during pregnancy, methyldopa, hydralazine, and labetalol are preferred agents because of more extensive experience with these agents in the pregnant patient. *Angiotensin-converting enzyme (ACE) inhibitors and angiotensin receptor blockers are contraindicated in pregnant patients.*

Pulmonary Hypertension

The primary care provider should be suspicious of this condition in patients with symptoms of syncope, fatigue, and dyspnea on exertion, particularly if the cardiac examination demonstrates a right ventricular heave, a loud P2, and murmurs of tricuspid and pulmonic insufficiency. The diagnosis usually can be confirmed by cardiac echocardiography.

Patients with pulmonary hypertension have a high maternal mortality rate of 40% to 50%. Therefore, patients with pulmonary hypertension should be strongly counseled against pregnancy. Patients with pulmonary hypertension who do become pregnant should be counseled that they are at high maternal risk if they carry through the pregnancy and should be referred to high-risk obstetricians.

Such patients who choose to continue their pregnancy should be treated with activity restriction and should be hospitalized at 28 to 30 weeks of gestation. Anticoagulation with subcutaneous heparin may be considered to reduce thromboembolic risk, although this is controversial. Anesthesia in patients with pulmonary hypertension should be administered only by specialized obstetric anesthesiologists. Future pregnancies should be discouraged with contraception (tubal ligation) counseling.

Acute Myocardial Infarction

Acute myocardial infarction is an unusual but potentially fatal complication seen in pregnancy. Although the usual etiologies of atherosclerosis, thrombosis, coronary artery aneurysm, and dissection have been reported, many women are found to have normal coronary anatomy at catheterization. Oral contraceptives, cocaine, and cigarette use are other risk factors seen in this patient population. Treatment of acute myocardial infarction is the same as in the nonpregnant patient, except that thrombolysis is not recommended. Primary angioplasty with pelvic shielding may be less risky to the fetus (although this may delay treatment of the mother and decrease the possible benefits of reperfusion therapy).

✪ CLINICAL PEARLS ✪

Diagnoses to consider in the pregnant or laboring patient with acute respiratory distress include pulmonary embolism from thromboembolic disease, amniotic fluid embolism, pneumomediastinum, and aspiration.

PREGNANCY AND VALVULAR HEART DISEASE

Mitral Stenosis

Mitral stenosis is the most common rheumatic valvular pathology in women of child-bearing age. The volume overloaded state and tachycardia of pregnancy can be poorly tolerated in patients with mitral stenosis who at baseline have a resting gradient across the mitral valve and rely on a long diastole to more completely empty the left atrium. These patients may decompensate with the development of sinus tachycardia or atrial fibrillation. In general, treatment is dictated primary by their New York Heart Association (NYHA) functional class. Asymptomatic or mildly symptomatic (NYHA Class I to II) patients should be treated with bed rest, salt restriction, treatment of concurrent infections, and judicial diuretic use to lower preload without compromising placental blood volume. Given these steps they usually will tolerate pregnancy and vaginal delivery well. Patients with more severe symptoms (NYHA Class III to IV, generally with a mitral valve area of less than 1.5 cm^2) generally require the earlier measures, along with hemodynamic monitoring during labor and delivery. Patients who develop heart failure despite these measures can be considered for balloon valvuloplasty or even mitral valve repair. Patients who develop atrial fibrillation should be rate controlled with a beta blocker or calcium antagonist prior to prompt cardioversion.

Aortic Stenosis

Aortic stenosis is usually the result of a congenital condition in child-bearing women. Most common is the scenario where the pregnant patient was born with a bicuspid aortic valve and then developed aortic stenosis. Clinically, patients can develop angina or heart failure during the hemodynamic changes of pregnancy. Surgical repair of significant aortic stenosis is recommended prior to contemplating pregnancy. The goal of management if patients with aortic stenosis who become pregnant should be to restrict activities and avoid hypovolemia. Refractory symptoms can be treated with surgical valve replacement or balloon valvotomy.

Mitral and Aortic Regurgitation

Mitral and aortic regurgitation are both well tolerated during pregnancy due to reduction of systemic vascular resistance and subsequent reduction of regurgitant volumes. Patients who develop symptoms of volume overload or heart failure can be treated with standard diuretics, digitalis, and vasodilators. Diuretics should be used cautiously to avoid excess volume depletion and subsequent reduced placental flow.

Prosthetic Valves

There are both advantages and disadvantages to both mechanical and bioprosthetic ("porcine" or "pig") valves with regard to pregnancy. Mechanical valves, although longer lasting, are associated during pregnancy with thrombotic complications and anticoagulation risks to the patient and fetus. Bioprosthetic valves do not expose the fetus to the risk of warfarin embryopathy, but they are not as durable as their mechanical counterparts. Patients with normally functioning prosthetic valves tolerate the hemodynamic changes of pregnancy without difficulty. Management of anticoagulation in patients with mechanical heart valves in discussed in the following section.

ANTICOAGULATION MANAGEMENT
WITH MECHANICAL HEART VALVES

In this section, possible strategies regarding anticoagulation decisions in patients with mechanical heart valves are discussed. Note, however, that anticoagulation decisions during pregnancy are complex, with significant and multiple risks to both the mother and fetus with either strategy. Strong consideration should be given to consulting specialists and thoroughly discussing the risks and benefits of anticoagulation strategies in patients who require anticoagulation during pregnancy.

Those patients with mechanical valves on warfarin anticoagulation should ideally stop warfarin prior to conception because of the risk of warfarin embryopathy to the developing fetus during the first trimester. In those women who are discovered to be pregnant, warfarin should be stopped immediately. In place of warfarin, subcutaneous heparin at an initial dose of 12,500 units b.i.d. should be initiated, then adjusted to maintain anticoagulation with a target-activated partial thromboplastin time (aPTT) of two to three times control. This should be titrated throughout the first trimester, with increasing heparin doses as plasma volume increases. An alternate to unfractured heparin may be the use of a low molecular weight heparin such as enoxaparin (Lovenox) or dalteparin (Fragmin).

✪   CLINICAL PEARLS   ✪

Warfarin embryopathy is the clinical syndrome of fetal microcephaly, optic atrophy, nasal bone hypoplasia, and epiphyseal stippling associated with maternal warfarin use during the first trimester.

Management During the Second and Third Trimesters

During the second and third trimesters, two management strategies can be considered. One strategy is to continue the patient on subcutaneous heparin therapy throughout the pregnancy. A second strategy would be to resume warfarin therapy until the middle of the third trimester, then again utilize subcutaneous heparin. Specialists differ on the relative risks of resuming warfarin therapy versus continuing heparin with regard to continued risks to the fetus and relative risks of thrombosis. A high-risk obstetric specialist should be consulted to discuss these risks with the primary care provider and the patient.

In those patients maintained on subcutaneous heparin therapy, the PTT should be monitored, as the dose of heparin necessary to maintain therapeutic PTT may increase during the pregnancy. Additionally, thrombocytopenia may develop with prolonged heparin use, and platelet counts should be monitored periodically.

Anticoagulation Around the Time of Delivery

As the expected delivery date approaches, the patient should be admitted to the hospital for conversion of warfarin or subcutaneous heparin to intravenous heparin. The target PTT with intravenous heparin should again be two to three times control. Heparin is stopped at labor onset and restarted 2 to 4 hours after delivery if there is no bleeding complication. Warfarin is resumed 24 hours after delivery, overlapped with heparin until the international normalized ratio is in the therapeutic range (2.5 to 3.5 in most cases, see Chapter 10). Warfarin can be continued in nursing mothers.

Enoxaparin

Enoxaparin (Lovenox) has been used in a small number of gravid patients successfully, but at this time there is no consensus on its routine use in the pregnant patient.

PREGNANCY AND CARDIAC ARRHYTHMIAS

Pregnancy is thought to increase the incidence of cardiac arrhythmias due to left atrial stretch from volume overload, increased sensitivity to catecholamines from gestational hormonal changes, and neurohumoral responses to psychological stressors.

Patients with cardiac arrhythmias should be instructed to avoid precipitating factors including tobacco, alcohol, caffeine, and illicit drugs. Medications with sympathomimetic activity, such as inhaled beta agonists and theophylline, should be avoided if possible.

In patients who develop reentrant supraventricular arrhythmias, vagal maneuvers should be attempted. Pharmacotherapy for supraventricular arrhythmias can include digoxin, adenosine, and beta blockers. Class IA agents (such as quinidine, procainamide, and disopyramide) can be considered for pregnant patients with ventricular arrhythmias; however, consultation with a specialist should be made before determining therapy for ventricular arrhythmias.

Cardioversion and Cardiac Arrest

Pregnant patients can be cardioverted successfully without adverse risk to the fetus. The risk of reduced placental flow during the tachyarrhythmia is higher than the risk of cardioversion. If the mother suffers full cardiopulmonary arrest, the uterus should be displaced from the vena cava during resuscitative measures. If the fetus is viable, emergency cesarean section should be performed after 15 minutes of unsuccessful maternal cardiopulmonary resuscitation.

PERIPARTUM CARDIOMYOPATHY

Peripartum cardiomyopathy is a poorly understood syndrome of congestive heart failure with ventricular dilation that is recognized in the third trimester of pregnancy or up to six months postpartum in patients without prior cardiac history.

Presentation and Diagnosis

Patients present with signs and symptoms of congestive heart failure, and the diagnosis is made by the demonstration of cardiomegaly and pulmonary vascular congestion by chest radiography and by four-chamber dilation with reduced systolic function by echocardiography. Peripartum cardiomyopathy is basically a diagnosis of exclusion, and other identifiable and reversible causes of cardiomyopathy (such as hypothyroidism or valvular heart disease) should be excluded. Consideration can be given to endomyocardial biopsy if there is a suspicion of a steroid-responsive process.

Management During Pregnancy

Medical therapy for peripartum cardiomyopathy generally is similar to that provided in nonpregnant patients. However, in those patients who are still pregnant, the combination of hydralazine and nitrate therapy should be used instead of ACE inhibitors (or angiotensin receptor blockers). Judicious diuretics and digoxin can be prescribed. Antiarrhythmic agents also may be considered, although some have potential adverse effects on the fetus. Patients should be instructed on salt restriction. In certain situations, bed rest should be prescribed and anticoagulation with heparin may be considered.

Delivery

Vaginal delivery often is tolerated well in the compensated patient. The patients should deliver in the lateral decubitus position. Pressure monitoring with a Swan-Ganz catheter should be performed by a specialist in the pregnant patient with decompensated heart failure unresponsive to appropriate management.

Postpartum Considerations

Long-term prognosis is not predictable at the time of presentation in patients with postpartum cardiomyopathy, but patients with persistent cardiomegaly 1 year after delivery do poorly. Patients with refractory heart failure after pregnancy would be candidates for assist devices as bridges to cardiac transplantation. Although reversal of ventricular dysfunction does occur in some patients, these patients nonetheless are at risk of developing recurrent myopathy with future pregnancies and should be strongly discouraged from having further pregnancies.

⟡ CLINICAL PEARLS ⟡

The use of tocolytic therapy to prolong gestation and allow fetal lung maturation has been associated with the development of maternal noncardiogenic pulmonary edema. This condition can be distinguished from peripartum cardiomyopathy by the finding of normal left ventricular function on cardiac echocardiogram. Treatment consists of termination of the agent, supplemental oxygen, and diuresis.

CARDIOVASCULAR DRUGS IN PREGNANCY

Any cardiovascular drugs used during pregnancy may potentially have effects on the fetus. The risk of fetal complications must be weighed against maternal benefit. The Food and Drug Administration categorizes the potential risk to the fetus of drugs based on available animal and human data. Drugs are categorized as pregnancy category A, B, C, D, or X. In general, drugs categorized as "A" or "B" are considered relatively safe and efficacious in pregnancy. Drugs categorized as "D" have been shown clearly to pose a risk to the fetus and should be avoided if possible. Drugs categorized as "X" are contraindicated during pregnancy. The classification of selected cardiovascular medications are listed in Table 13.1.

ENDOCARDITIS PROPHYLAXIS

The American Heart Association recommends endocarditis prophylaxis for patients with prosthetic valves or surgical systemic-to-pulmonic shunt undergoing vaginal delivery (Table 13.2). However, many cardiologists use prophylaxis for all congenital lesions except atrial septal defect and corrected patent ductus arteriosus during vaginal delivery. Prophylaxis is not recommended for elective cesarean deliveries.

All patients with prosthetic valves should receive endocarditis prophylaxis (gentamicin/ampicillin) at the time of vaginal delivery. Prophylaxis is not currently recommended by the American Heart Association

TABLE 13.2. *Suggested regimens for endocarditis prophylaxis in pregnant patients undergoing vaginal delivery*[a]

Patient risk	Drug and dosage regimen
High-risk patients[b]	
• Standard regimen	Ampicillin 2 g i.v. or i.m. plus gentamicin 1.5 mg/kg (not to exceed 120 mg) i.v. 30 min prior to delivery; then 6 h later give either ampicillin 1 g i.m. or i.v. or amoxicillin 1 g p.o.
• Penicillin-allergic patients	Vancomycin 1 gm i.v. over 1–2 h plus gentamicin 1.5 mg/kg (not to exceed 120 mg) i.v. or i.m. within 30 min of delivery
Moderate-risk patients[c]	
• Standard regimen	Amoxicillin 2 gm p.o. 1 h prior to delivery or ampicillin 2 gm i.m./i.v. within 30 min of delivery
• Penicillin-allergic patients	Vancomycin 1 gm i.v. over 1–2 h completed within 30 min of delivery

[a] Prophylaxis in moderate-risk patients is at the practitioner's discretion.
[b] Includes patients with prosthetic cardiac valves, history of previous bacterial endocarditis, complex cyanotic congenital heart disease, or surgically constructed systemic pulmonary shunts or conduits.
[c] Includes patients with most other congenital cardiac malformations (other than above), acquired valvular dysfunction (e.g., rheumatic heart disease), hypertrophic cardiomyopathy, mitral valve prolapse with valvular regurgitation, and/or thickened leaflets.

in uncomplicated cesarean delivery, although many obstetricians and cardiologists have a low threshold for using antibiotic prophylaxis in the patient with prosthetic valves, however, for cesarean section (see Table 13.2).

For the purposes of deciding which pregnant patients with cardiovascular disease should receive endocarditis prophylaxis, patients can be classified as either high risk or moderate risk. High-risk patients include those with:

- Prosthetic cardiac valves (including bioprosthetic and homograft valves)
- History of previous bacterial endocarditis
- Complex cyanotic congenital heart disease
- Surgically constructed systemic-to-pulmonic shunts or conduits.

Patients considered to be at moderate risk include those with:

- Most other congenital cardiac malformations (other than above)
- Acquired valvular dysfunction (e.g., rheumatic heart disease)
- Hypertrophic cardiomyopathy
- Mitral valve prolapse with valvular regurgitation and/or thickened leaflets.

SUMMARY

Women at high risk for maternal or fetal mortality should be counseled before pregnancy is contemplated, and corrective procedures should be planned accordingly. Treatment during pregnancy should focus on both maternal and fetal well-being, with attendant risk-to-benefit assessments at each encounter. Many cardiac conditions can be treated similarly with medications used in nonpregnant patients; however, ACE inhibitors, angiotensin receptor blockers, amiodarone, and warfarin may pose unacceptable risks to the fetus. Certain conditions warrant endocarditis prophylaxis during delivery.

14

What Primary Care Providers Need to Know About Cardiac Catheterization, Angioplasty, and Coronary Stents

M. Nadir Ali and Glenn N. Levine

Baylor College of Medicine, Cardiac Catheterization Laboratory, Houston V. A. Medical Center, Houston, Texas 77030

More than 1 million patients in the United States alone undergo cardiac catheterization and percutaneous revascularization (percutaneous transluminal coronary angioplasty [PTCA], stents, etc.). While you will not be performing the actual procedure, you will nevertheless be intimately involved in the care of such patients, from deciding which patients to refer to a cardiologist for cardiac catheterization through checking up and following the patient after the catheterization or angioplasty. In this chapter, information useful to primary care providers regarding cardiac catheterization, balloon angioplasty, and coronary stenting is discussed.

CARDIAC CATHETERIZATION

Indications

The primary indication for cardiac catheterization is to determine coronary anatomy to facilitate revascularization decisions. Although opinion differs, generally accepted indications for cardiac catheterization can include:

- Anginal symptoms not controlled with medical therapy
- Markedly positive stress test
- Unstable angina refractory to medical therapy
- Postmyocardial infarction angina or positive predischarge exercise test
- Moderately or severely depressed ejection fraction when coronary artery disease is the suspected etiology
- Symptomatic valvular disease (particularly if surgery is being considered).

During the cardiac catheterization procedure, a pencil-sized plastic sheath is inserted into the femoral artery. A coronary catheter is then threaded through the sheath, up the descending aorta, around the aortic arch, down the ascending aorta, and engaged into a coronary ostium. Iodine-based dye is injected as cineangiography is performed in multiple different projections. The entire process can take as little as 15 minutes or as long as 1 hour. A typical angiogram, this one showing a tight stenosis of the right coronary artery, is shown in Fig. 14.1A.

Complications

Although cardiac catheterization is regarded as a generally safe procedure, complications occasionally occur, and the primary care provider should be aware of several issues. An increased incidence of dye-allergic reactions has been noted in patients who are allergic to shellfish. Thus, patients should be questioned if they have such allergic reactions or if they have had allergic reactions to dye in the past. Such patients need to be pretreated with steroids.

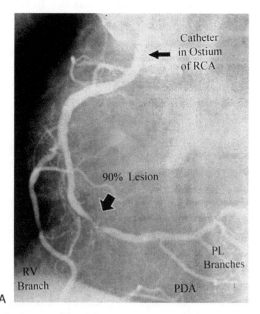

FIG. 14.1. A: Angiogram of the right coronary artery (RCA) showing a 90% lesion. RV branch, right ventricular branch.

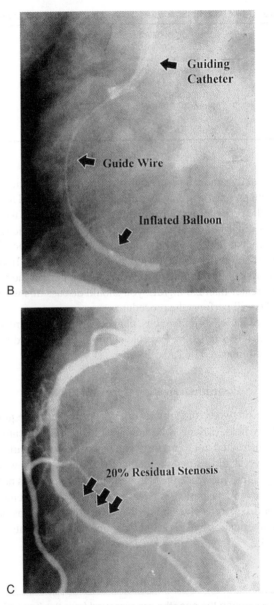

FIG. 14.1. B: During angioplasty, a guidewire is threaded across the lesion. Then a small balloon is delivered over this guidewire to the lesion and is inflated to several atmospheres of pressure. **C**: Only a mild residual stenosis remains at the site of the treated lesion.

TABLE 14.1. *Complications associated with cardiac catheterization*

Local complications at vascular access site
  • Bleeding (hematoma)
  • Infection
  • Vascular damage
Dye-induced allergic reaction
Dye-induced renal failure
Myocardial infarction
Stroke
Death

The risk of dye-induced renal failure is higher in diabetic patients and in those with preexisting renal insufficiency. Because good hydration status before the procedure is the only thing that can decrease the chances of developing renal failure after a catheterization, some practitioners will admit patients at high risk of dye-induced renal failure the night before the catheterization to hydrate them before the procedure. If your patient is at higher risk of developing renal failure, particularly if the baseline creatinine is greater than 2.0 mg/dL, you should discuss this with the cardiologist who will perform the procedure.

The risk of major complications, namely, heart attack, stroke, or death, is approximately 1 in 1,000. Possible complications of cardiac catheterization are summarized in Table 14.1.

Postcatheterization Care and Follow-up

Because the site where the femoral artery was punctured requires several days to fully heal, patients who have just had a cardiac catheterization should be instructed not to perform any heavy exertion (particularly lifting) for several days after the catheterization. Patients who undergo "same day caths," in which the catheterization procedure is performed as an outpatient, and the patient is released to go home at the end of the day, should not drive themselves home that day. Important considerations in the precatheterization and pericatheterization care of patients are outlined in Table 14.2.

✪ CLINICAL PEARLS ✪

Occasionally, when the sheaths are removed from the femoral artery, the puncture site in the artery does not seal properly and a pseudoaneurysm can develop. The findings of a pulsatile area and a bruit at the site of sheath insertion suggest the presence of a pseudoaneurysm, and an ultrasound test should be ordered. Larger pseudoaneurysms (larger than 1 × 1 cm) usually need to be treated with surgery.

TABLE 14.2. *Considerations in, and care of, patients undergoing cardiac catheterization*

1. Evaluate the need for cardiac catheterization
2. Discuss the procedure and possible complications
3. Determine if the patient is allergic to dye or shellfish, and thus if he or she needs to be premedicated with steroids
4. Evaluate if the patient is at increased risk for dye-induced renal failure
5. Check the patient's groin and peripheral pulses post procedure for signs of bleeding, infection, or vascular damage
6. Remind the patient not to perform any heavy exertion for several days after the catheterization

PERCUTANEOUS TRANSLUMINAL CORONARY ANGIOPLASTY

Procedure

In coronary angioplasty, a guiding catheter is first engaged in the target coronary artery. An ultrathin guidewire then is threaded across the stenosis to be treated. A thin balloon is in turn threaded over the guidewire and across the lesion, and the balloon is inflated to several atmospheres of pressure. Inflation of the balloon serves to open the artery both by stretching the artery wider and by "compressing" the plaque that is causing the stenosis. The procedure is demonstrated in Figs. 14.1B and 14.1C. The PTCA procedure is successful in dilating the coronary lesion in more than 90% of cases.

Complications

Complications of PTCA include those associated with cardiac catheterization. Additionally, when the angioplasty balloon is inflated, it may occasionally "rip" the artery, leading to arterial dissection. If this dissection is serious enough, it can obstruct blood flow down the artery. Because of this, there is an approximately 1–2% chance of the patient suffering an acute myocardial infarction or requiring emergency bypass surgery. The risk of dying during PTCA is approximately 1%.

Indications

As with cardiac catheterization, there is some variability in which patients practitioners believe should undergo PTCA. Although no definitive recommendations can be given, patients who it is generally agreed are reasonable candidates for referral for PTCA include:

• Patients with stable angina and single vessel coronary artery disease whose symptoms are not easily controlled with medications, who do not tolerate their medications, or who desire to pursue a moderately or intensely active lifestyle

- Patients with multivessel coronary artery disease and significant symptoms who desire to be treated with PTCA instead of bypass surgery
- Patients with unstable angina who are found at cardiac catheterization to have a lesion amenable to PTCA
- Patients with acute myocardial infarction who can be quickly triaged to a catheterization team and laboratory that is ready to perform PTCA.

Restenosis

In approximately one third of patients treated with balloon angioplasty, the stenosis will recur, a phenomenon known as restenosis. Restenosis usually occurs 1 to 6 months after the angioplasty procedure, with patients most commonly presenting with recurrent angina. Restenosis usually can be treated with repeat angioplasty. In some cases, restenosis may require bypass surgery.

Care of the Patient After Percutaneous Transluminal Coronary Angioplasty

Patients who undergo PTCA usually are discharged 1 or 2 days after the procedure. As with patients who have undergone cardiac catheterization, patients who have undergone PTCA should be instructed not to perform any heavy exertion (particularly lifting) for several days after the PTCA. In general, patients are advised not to drive for 1 to 2 days after the PTCA. Patients usually can resume normal activities, including returning to work and sexual activities (something all patients and their spouses worry about but never ask about), within 1 week.

Coronary Stents

Over the last several years, stainless steel coronary stents have been increasingly utilized. Advantages of stents include the facts that implantation of stents can decrease acute complication rates (particularly the need for emergency bypass surgery) and decrease the incidence of restenosis to approximately 1 in 5 patients.

Treatment with a potent antiplatelet agent in addition to aspirin therapy has been shown to decrease the incidence of stent thrombosis (which can occur in the first several weeks after stent implantation). In the past, the potent antiplatelet agent ticlopidine (Ticlid), administered 250 mg by p.o. b.i.d., was used. More recently, more physicians are utilizing clopidogrel (Plavix), administered 75 mg p.o. qd. Most physicians who implant stents will treat patients with ticlopidine or clopidogrel for 2 to 4 weeks after stent implantation.

❖ CLINICAL PEARLS ❖

Reversible neutropenia occurs in 1% to 2% of patients treated with ticlopidine. Therefore, a white blood cell (WBC) count should be obtained after 2 weeks of therapy in patients treated with ticlopidine (it is not necessary to monitor WBC counts in patients on clopidogrel). Also, because treatment with either of these potent antiplatelet agents is only necessary for several weeks, and as the risk of neutropenia with ticlopidine increases over time, patients should only be treated for a total of 2 to 4 weeks (as prescribed by the interventional cardiologist). Primary care providers should ensure that these medications are not inadvertently renewed beyond 2 to 4 weeks. Finally, note that during this time (and thereafter) patients should still be being treated with aspirin.

Two questions that often come up in patients treated with coronary stents are (i) what are the recommendations regarding endocarditis prophylaxis and (ii) can patients undergo an magnetic resonance imaging (MRI). Unfortunately, there are neither hard data nor firm recommendations regarding the answer to either of these questions. One reasonable approach would be to use antibiotic prophylaxis, when indicated, for the first 3 or 4 weeks after stent implantation until the stent has become endothelialized (the process whereby a layer of endothelial cells grows over and covers the metal stent). Once the stent has become endothelialized, antibiotic prophylaxis probably is not necessary (though again there are no data regarding this).

In patients in whom MRI is being contemplated, the general feeling is that, if possible, elective MRIs should be deferred for about 4 weeks after stent implantation. In patients who must undergo urgent MRI (such as for a central nervous system catastrophe), it generally is recommended that they should undergo MRI when and as clinically necessary.

Care of Patients Treated with Platelet IIb/IIIa Receptor Inhibitors

Platelet IIb/IIIa receptor inhibitors are a new class of potent antiplatelet agents that have been shown to decrease complication rates during PTCA and coronary stent procedures. These agents are currently utilized in more than half of all percutaneous interventions. Three agents currently are being utilized. After procedures in which any of these agents are given, heparin should not be given (or continued), as this can increase bleeding complications (although there may be rare cases where the interventionalist does continue some form of anticoagulation). Considerations specific to each agent are as follows:

Abciximab (ReoPro):
- 250 μg/kg i.v. bolus (usually given in the catheterization laboratory), then continue infusion at 0.125 μg/kg/min (up to maximum of 10 μg/

min) for 12 hours postprocedure (note that dose is in micrograms, not milligrams)
- Check platelet count (due to small risk of thrombocytopenia) 2 to 4 hours after therapy is initiated and the following morning; discontinue infusion if platelet count drops to less than 100,000/mm³.

Eptifibatide (Integrilin):
- A bolus dose of 180 µg/kg is given (usually in the catheterization laboratory), then continue infusion at 2 µg/kg/min for 20 to 24 hours postprocedure. Maintenance dose should be adjusted in patients with renal insufficiency (note that dose is in micrograms, not milligrams).

Tirofiban (Aggrastat):
- An initial infusion of 0.4 µg/kg/min for 30 minutes is given (usually started in the catheterization laboratory), then continue infusion at 0.1 µg/kg/min for 12 to 24 hours postprocedure (note that dose is in micrograms, not milligrams). Bolus and maintenance dose should be adjusted in patients with renal insufficiency.
- Check platelet count (due to small risk of thrombocytopenia) within 6 hours after therapy is initiated and the following morning; discontinue infusion if platelet count drops to less than 90,000/mm³.

Evaluation of the Patient with Recurrent Chest Pain

In patients who develop recurrent chest pain in the first 6 months after PTCA, the likely cause is restenosis. Noninvasive testing of patients with recurrent chest pain after PTCA, including exercise treadmill testing, exercise or dobutamine echocardiography, and nuclear imaging studies, generally are not sensitive or specific enough to confidently rule in or rule out the occurrence of restenosis. The most prudent course of action in these patients is referral for cardiac catheterization to assess if restenosis has occurred.

Considerations in, and care of, patients treated with PTCA or stents are listed in Table 14.3.

SUMMARY

Important issues of which the primary care provider should be aware in the precatheterization care of patients include discussing the procedure and risks with the patient, evaluating the risk of dye-induced renal failure, discussing the need for precatheterization hydration with the cardiologist who will perform the procedure, checking if the patient is allergic to dye or shellfish and if he or she needs to be premedicated with steroids, and adjusting and/or holding diabetic medications.

TABLE 14.3. *Considerations in, and care of, patients treated with PTCA or stents*

1. Evaluate if the procedure is actually indicated
2. Make sure the patient understands the procedure and possible complications
3. Remind patients who have undergone PTCA not to perform any heavy exertion (particularly lifting) for several days after the PTCA
4. Advise patients not to drive for a day or two after the PTCA
5. Advise most patients (except those with complicated hospital courses) that they can resume normal activities, including returning to work and sexual activities, within about 1 wk
6. Check the patient's groin and peripheral pulses post procedure for signs of bleeding, infection, or vascular damage
7. Verify with patients treated with stents that they are taking either ticlopidine or plavix for 2 to 4 wks after the stent procedure, and that if on ticlopidine a white blood cell count was or will be performed after 2 wk of therapy.
8. Consider antibiotic prophylaxis, when indicated, for the first 3 to 4 wk after stent implantation
9. In patients with recurrent chest pain, particularly within the first 6 mo after PTCA or stenting, consider referral for cardiac catheterization

PTCA, percutaneous transluminal coronary angioplasty.

Initial activity restrictions and the subsequent time course for resumption of normal activities should be discussed with the patient. In patients treated with coronary stent implantation, the practitioner should verify that the patient is taking ticlopidine or clopidogrel for the prescribed 2–4 weeks after the procedure. In patients who develop recurrent chest pain after PTCA or stenting, referral for cardiac catheterization should be considered.

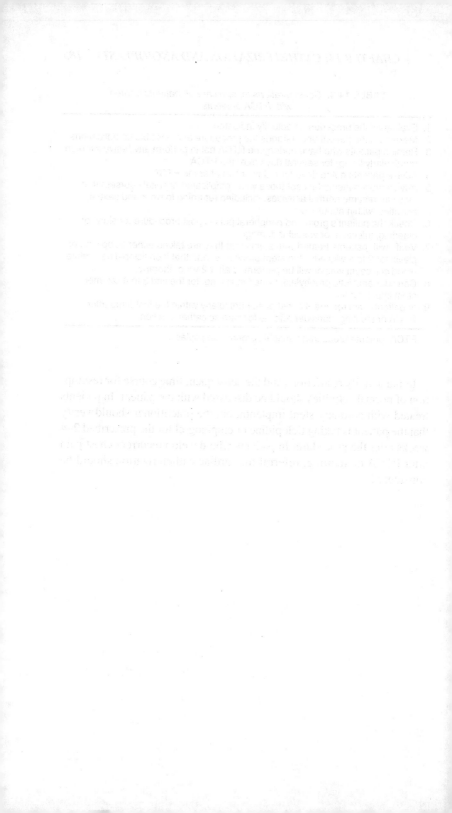

15

Caring for Patients with Pacemakers and Implantable Cardioverter-Defibrillators

Karen M. Belco

Cardiology Associates of Lubbock, Lubbock, Texas 79410

Patients with pacemakers and implantable cardioverter-defibrillators (ICDs) require specialized follow-up. Although this additional specialized care generally is provided by trained electrophysiologist "device specialists," the primary care provider is likely to be confronted with increasing numbers of patients with these devices as the population continues to age. Further, because the primary care provider often will be the health care provider following the patient most closely, he or she should be familiar with the follow-up that the patient should be receiving. The primary care provider should have a basic understanding of the many factors in the environment that can impact on pacemakers and ICDs. In this chapter, the standard of care for patients with pacemakers and ICDs, as well as the special precautions that are required for patients with pacemakers and ICDs, are reviewed. The psychological impact on the patient of these devices is discussed in terms of what the primary care provider should be aware of as well as how to deal with this issue.

WHAT PRIMARY CARE PROVIDERS SHOULD KNOW ABOUT PACEMAKERS

Pacemakers need to be checked at regular intervals to ensure appropriate functioning of both the pacemaker generator and the pacemaker leads. However, many patients often are lost to follow-up. The primary care physician should always check with the patient that he or she has returned to the specialist for appropriate testing.

Frequency of Pacemaker Follow-up

The frequency of pacemaker follow-up currently is determined by the Medicare guidelines for routine follow-up. The goals of follow-up are to determine if (i) the pacemaker needs to be adjusted in the months after implantation and (ii) the battery of the pacemaker is wearing out (the average life of an implanted pacemaker is approximately 5 to 8 years).

Transtelephonic monitoring for most pacemakers generally should be performed:

- Every 2 weeks the first month
- Every 4 weeks during months 2 through 6
- Every eight weeks during months 7 through 36
- Every 4 weeks from month 37 until end of service.

✪ CLINICAL PEARLS ✪

During clinic visits, pacing thresholds (the amount of electrical energy required to stimulate myocardial contraction) are performed and adjustments are made as needed to ensure the safe functioning of the pacemaker and that the life of the battery is preserved.

Threshold testing (which requires a visit to an electrophysiologic device specialist) in the outpatient setting should be performed:

- Twice in the first 6 months following pacemaker implantation
- Every 6 months thereafter.

Antibiotic Prophylaxis

Antibiotic prophylaxis is not necessary for patients with pacemakers.

INITIAL STEPS TO TAKE WHEN PACEMAKER MALFUNCTION IS SUSPECTED

Electrocardiography

When confronted with the question of whether the pacemaker is functioning properly, it is appropriate to obtain a 12-lead electrocardiogram with a rhythm strip. If the primary care provider observes pacemaker "spikes" on the electrocardiogram without a p wave or QRS complex following it, this suggests that the pacemaker is not capturing properly. If the pacemaker spikes are not "inhibited" by p waves or QRS complexes (i.e., the pacemaker "fires" despite the the presence of a native P wave or QRS complex), this suggests that the pacemaker is not sensing appropriately.

If the paced QRS complexes do not have a left bundle branch morphology, this suggests that the pacemaker lead has migrated and is no longer stimulating the right ventricle.

Chest Radiography

Routine chest x-ray films for patients with pacemakers are seldom helpful, and they are not necessary in the routine management of patients with pacemakers, except when troubleshooting pacemaker malfunction is necessary.

Referral

In patients in whom there remains a question of pacemaker functioning, referral to a device specialist is appropriate.

✪ CLINICAL PEARLS ✪

Patients should be reminded to carry with them *at all times* a card (given to them at the time of implantation) containing important information regarding the pacemaker.

WHAT THE PRIMARY CARE PROVIDER NEEDS TO KNOW ABOUT IMPLANTABLE CARDIOVERTER-DEFIBRILLATORS (ICDs)

Follow-up

Guidelines for follow-up of ICDs are less specific than for pacemakers. In general, a routine evaluation is done every 3 to 4 months. It is performed more frequently if the patient is having tachyarrhythmias and receiving pharmacologic therapy for these arrhythmias. During routine clinic visits, the device specialist will retrieve diagnostic arrhythmia data from the ICD itself. This information is reviewed and correlated with the patient's symptoms to evaluate the type and frequency of arrhythmias and the appropriateness of the therapies that are being delivered. The new generation of ICDs offers dual and single chamber bradycardia pacing support. As with permanent pacemakers, pacing and sensing thresholds are performed for the pacemaking aspects of the ICD. Battery voltages are monitored to ensure proper functioning of the device. Transtelephonic monitoring of ICDs is not routinely performed.

What to Do When a Patient's Implantable Cardioverter-Defibrillator Discharges

Given the complexity of the current ICDs and the complexity of the arrhythmias of these patients, as well as the potential for untoward clinical outcomes in ICD patients, the primary care provider should always promptly refer these patients to a cardiovascular device specialist or to a cardiologist who is familiar with these devices.

Antibiotic Prophylaxis

As with pacemakers, antibiotic prophylaxis is not necessary for patients with implanted cardiac devices.

EFFECTS OF COMMON ANTIARRHYTHMIC DRUGS ON PACING AND DEFIBRILLATION THRESHOLDS

Although the use of antiarrhythmic drugs is common in patients with cardiac devices, there are several considerations to keep in mind when using these agents.

Effects of Antiarrhythmic Agents on Pacing Thresholds

Type IA antiarrhythmics, such as procainamide and disopyramide, can increase pacing thresholds, especially with higher doses. Type IC drugs, such as propafenone and flecainide, are known to elevate thresholds. Amiodarone has been associated with increased pacing thresholds. Therefore, if antiarrhythmic agents are begun or the dose of the agent is changed, the primary care provider should discuss this with the device specialist whether the patient needs to be seen and whether pacing thresholds need to be rechecked.

Effects of Antiarrhythmic Agents on Defibrillation Thresholds

Some drugs, such as amiodarone and verapamil, can have an adverse effect on defibrillation thresholds. In contrast, sotalol lowers defibrillation thresholds. The primary care provider should always refer these patients to a device specialist to evaluate pacing thresholds after these drugs are initiated or if the drug dose is altered to assure the safety margins of programmed energy outputs.

ENVIRONMENTAL INTERFERENCE OF CARDIAC DEVICES

Electromagnetic Noise

Environmental electromagnetic noise signals (such as those generated by car engines or heavy industrial equipment) may interfere with normal pacemaker function by inappropriately inhibiting the pacemaker, although most newer pacemakers are designed to deal with this occurrence. However, electromagnetic interference also can cause a mode change in the pacemaker that will need reprogramming to restore original values. Therefore, in patients who have been exposed to electromagnetic interference, consider referral to a device specialist to check that the pacemaker is still operating in the correct programmed mode.

Electrocautery

The surgical use of electrocautery devices in patients with pacemakers or ICDs requires special monitoring. Electrocautery most frequently uses radiofrequency energy delivered between the pencil electrode and a grounding plate on the skin. The electrical interference generated by the electrocautery can inhibit implanted pacemakers and ICDs if either of these devices falsely detects the electrical interference as an intrinsic heart rhythm. This may cause asystole and/or hemodynamic compromise in a patient who is dependent on the pacemaker. Therefore, in patients who are pacemaker dependent, consideration should be given to program the pacemaker in an asynchronous mode to avoid asystole.

A magnet may be placed over the pacemaker to convert the pacemaker to an asynchronous mode; however, some devices have a finite number of asynchronous pulses delivered before reverting back to the programmed mode. Moreover, manufacturers do not recommend this practice because application of a magnet may cause the program to reprogram itself. Additionally, electrocautery can set the pacemaker to "back-up" mode, which will require postoperative reprogramming. In general, device specialists usually do not reprogram pacemakers prior to surgery. Instead, they instruct the surgeon to use short electrocautery bursts of less than 2 seconds. Less common problems seen with electrocautery include pacemaker circuit damage, elevated thresholds, and rate responsive pacemakers pacing at the upper rate limit.

Patients with ICDs should be referred to a device specialist to have what is called "tachycardia detection" disabled, because the ICD may interpret the cautery signal as a tachycardia and inappropriately deliver antitachycardia therapy to the patient. The electrocardiographic rhythm and pacemaker function should be monitored carefully during electrocautery application, and ideally the device should be evaluated postoperatively by a trained device specialist.

If a patient with an ICD requires emergency surgery, the device specialist should be called. If the specialist is not available, one can call the manufacturer's representative for instructions on how to manage the patient. There is a number to call to contact the representative on the patient's ICD identification card.

Magnetic Resonance Imaging

Magnetic resonance imaging can have various temporary adverse effects on cardiac devices. Therefore, it is recommended that people with implanted cardiac devices avoid undergoing magnetic resonance imaging.

Radiation

Routine diagnostic x-rays have no effect on pacemaker or ICD function. However, therapeutic radiation, such as is used in the treatment of malignancies, can damage both pacemakers and ICDs. The damage to these devices may be so severe that they have to be replaced. A device specialist should be consulted prior to initiation of radiation therapy. The radiation therapist should be instructed to ensure adequate shielding of the devices to minimize radiation exposure. The patient who is pacemaker dependent should undergo continuous electrocardiographic monitoring during radiation therapy.

Lithotripsy

Lithotripsy generally is considered safe in patients with pacemakers. However, some pacemakers with piezoelectric sensors can be damaged if they are placed directly in the pathway of the lithotriptor output pulse. If the patient has a rate sensing pacemaker, the rate adaptation should be programmed off prior to the procedure. It is suggested that dual chamber pacemakers be reprogrammed to a single chamber (VVI) to avoid having the lithotriptor trigger the atrial pulse. Patients with cardiac devices implanted in the abdomen should avoid the lithotripsy procedure. Finally, pacemakers should be evaluated postprocedure to ensure proper functioning.

Transcutaneous Electric Nerve Stimulation

Transcutaneous electric nerve stimulation usually can be used safely with bipolar cardiac devices. However, some (older) unipolar pacemakers with a high sensitivity may be inhibited. Transcutaneous electric nerve stimulation near the pacemaker should be avoided.

Cardioversion/Defibrillation

External transthoracic cardioversion/defibrillation can damage pacemakers and ICDs. However, these devices now have protective filtering to prevent high-energy currents from being conducted to the myocardium through the intracardiac leads. High-energy currents that are delivered through the leads can cause myocardial damage with resultant loss of sensing and capture.

When cardioversion of defibrillation is necessary, place the defibrillator paddles as far away from the device as possible *(the paddles should never be placed over the device!)*. Use the lowest possible energy to convert the rhythm.

The most common problems associated with external defibrillation are reversion of pacemakers to back-up mode and triggering of the end-of-life indicator. Accordingly, a device specialist should be available afterward for threshold testing and device reprogramming when elective cardioversions are planned, or should be consulted immediately afterward if urgent or emergent cardioversion or defibrillation is performed.

Cellular Telephones

Cellular telephones can interfere temporarily with the proper functioning of cardiac devices. In this regard, digital phones are more likely to cause interference than are analog signal phones. Instruct patients to keep the phone a minimum distance of 6 inches away from the device to minimize problems.

External Pulse Counters

External devices for counting heart rate are used commonly during exercise, particularly in cardiac rehabilitation programs. Some external heart rate monitors come with warnings to contact a physician prior to use. Although pacemakers do not appear to interfere with external heart rate monitors, they may cause the pulse counter to render false readings because the pulse counter may count both the pacemaker pulse and the patient's QRS, thereby recording a heart rate that is double the actual heart rate.

Arc Welding

Arc welding is strictly contraindicated in patients with cardiac devices because there is a significant risk of pacemaker inhibition.

Metal Detectors

Metal detectors such as those found in airports do not affect cardiac devices significantly. Although there may be inhibition of one or two paced beats in some (older unipolar) pacemakers, this is not likely to cause the patient any symptoms. Because most metal detectors are quite sensitive, it is more than likely that patients with pacemakers and ICDs will set off the metal detector alarm. Therefore, patients should carry an identification card identifying the implanted device. *Be sure that patients who you are following know that handheld wand metal detectors can cause a problem with detection of the electrocardiographic signal detected by the pacemaker or ICD and can cause false signals and thus should not be used near the device.*

Antitheft Scanners

Antitheft devices commonly seen at department store entrances do not adversely affect devices, except for a one-beat inhibition of some (older unipolar) pacemakers.

⟡ CLINICAL PEARLS ⟡

Most electrical equipment found in the home, such as microwave ovens, electric shavers, electric blankets, and drills will not cause damage to cardiac devices, particularly the newer devices.

PSYCHOLOGICAL IMPACT
OF CARDIAC DEVICE IMPLANTATION

Many patients have difficulty accepting and/or adjusting to having an artificial device implanted in their body. Having a pacemaker or an ICD implanted is emotionally stressful to many patients, who do not like the idea of being dependent on a "machine" for sustaining their life. Moreover, many patients may lose their jobs because they have an implanted cardiac device (e.g., truck drivers, airline pilots, arc welders). The stress surrounding implantation of cardiac devices has been heightened as hospital lengths of stay have become progressively shorter. The shorter hospital stay often does not allow time for the patient to have as much contact with health care professionals, who might be able to provide additional education and counseling and thereby help to minimize anxiety.

The primary care provider should be aware that patient and family education can hep alleviate many of the fears that patients and families have. Psychological counseling of the patient and family may be necessary in some cases. It is important that instructions given to the patient and family are consistently the same from all members of the health care team, so that patients and families do not get "mixed messages."

SUMMARY

Pacemakers and ICDs need to be checked at regular intervals. The primary care provider should review with the patient if he/she is being followed-up appropriately with the device specialist. Antiarrhythmic drugs can affect pacing and defibrillation thresholds, and the addition of new antiarrhythmic agents or changes in the doses of current antiarrhythmic agents should be discussed with a device specialist. External factors that can have an adverse impact on the pacemaker or ICD include electromechanical noise, electrocautery, radiation therapy, cardioversion/ defibrillation, cellular phones, and arc welding. Many patients have psychological issues with having an artificial device in their body, and the primary care provider should be alert to such signs and be aware that patient and family education can help alleviate many such issues.

Subject Index

Numbers followed by the letter f indicate figures; numbers followed by the letter t indicate tables.